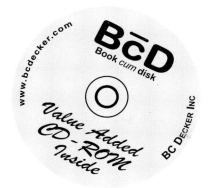

CRANIAL NERVES

in health and disease

SECOND EDITION

LINDA WILSON-PAUWELS, AOCA, BScAAM, MEd, EdD
Professor and Director
Biomedical Communications, Department of Surgery
Faculty of Medicine
University of Toronto
Toronto, Ontario

ELIZABETH J. AKESSON, BA, MSc
Assistant Professor (Emerita)
Department of Anatomy
Faculty of Medicine
University of British Columbia
Vancouver, British Columbia

PATRICIA A. STEWART, BSc, MSc, PhD
Professor
Anatomy, Department of Surgery
Faculty of Medicine
University of Toronto
Toronto, Ontario

SIÂN D. SPACEY, BSc, MBBS, FRCPC
Assistant Professor
Neurology, Department of Medicine
Faculty of Medicine
University of British Columbia
Vancouver, British Columbia

2002
BC Decker Inc
Hamilton • London

BC Decker Inc
20 Hughson Street South
P.O. Box 620, LCD 1
Hamilton, Ontario L8N 3K7
Tel: 905-522-7017; 800-568-7281
Fax: 905-522-7839
E-mail: info@bcdecker.com
Web site: www.bcdecker.com

02 03 04 05 /PC/ 9 8 7 6 5 4 3 2 1

ISBN 1-55009-164-6
Printed in Canada

Sales and Distribution

United States
BC Decker Inc
P.O. Box 785
Lewiston, NY 14092-0785
Tel: 905-522-7017; 800-568-7281
Fax: 905-522-7839
E-mail: info@bcdecker.com
Web site: www.bcdecker.com

Canada
BC Decker Inc
20 Hughson Street South
P.O. Box 620, LCD 1
Hamilton, Ontario L8N 3K7
Tel: 905-522-7017; 800-568-7281
Fax: 905-522-7839
E-mail: info@bcdecker.com
Web site: www.bcdecker.com

Foreign Rights
John Scott & Company
International Publishers' Agency
P.O., Box 878
Kimberton, PA 19442
Tel: 610-827-1640
Fax: 610-827-1671
E-mail: jsco@voicenet.com

Japan
Igaku-Shoin Ltd.
Foreign Publications Department
3-24-17 Hongo
Bunkyo-ku, Tokyo, Japan 113-8719
Tel: 3 3817 5680
Fax: 3 3815 6776
E-mail: fd@igaku.shoin.co.jp

U.K., Europe, Scandinavia, Middle East
Elsevier Science
Customer Service Department
Foots Cray High Street
Sidcup, Kent
DA14 5HP, UK
Tel: 44 (0) 208 308 5760
Fax: 44 (0) 181 308 5702
E-mail: cservice@harcourt.com

Singapore, Malaysia, Thailand, Philippines, Indonesia, Vietnam, Pacific Rim, Korea
Elsevier Science Asia
583 Orchard Road
#09/01, Forum
Singapore 238884
Tel: 65-737-3593
Fax: 65-753-2145

Australia, New Zealand
Elsevier Science Australia
Customer Service Department
STM Division
Locked Bag 16
St. Peters, New South Wales, 2044
Australia
Tel: 61 02 9517-8999
Fax: 61 02 9517-2249
Email: stmp@harcourt.com.au
Web site: www.harcourt.com.au

Preface

The second edition of *Cranial Nerves* reflects the shift in teaching methods from didactic lectures to problem-based learning. The book has maintained the original approach of the first edition, that is, a blending of the neuro- and gross anatomy of the cranial nerves as seen through color-coded functional drawings of the pathways from the periphery of the body to the brain (sensory input) and from the brain to the periphery (motor output).

In this second edition, Dr. Siân Spacey, a neurologist, has joined the original three coauthors: Dr. Linda Wilson-Pauwels, Prof. Elizabeth Akesson, and Dr. Patricia Stewart. As a team, we have revised the original text and visual material, developed case history scenarios with guiding questions, and provided clinical testing scenarios for each nerve in both the text and on CD-ROM. The artwork is now full color and several concepts are animated on the CD-ROM.

The "Functional Combinations" chapter from the first edition has been removed, and nerves acting together have been moved to their appropriate chapters. Chapter 13, "Coordinated Eye Movements," highlights the three cranial nerves responsible for these important actions.

Cranial Nerves is still targeted to students of the health sciences (medicine, rehabilitation sciences, dentistry, pharmacy, speech pathology, audiology, nursing, physical and health education, and biomedical communications) who may be studying neuroanatomy and gross anatomy for the first time. We discovered that the first edition (printed in 1988) was a valuable quick reference for residents in neurology, neurosurgery, otolaryngology, and maxillofacial surgery; therefore, this second edition includes additional clinical material.

Linda Wilson-Pauwels
Elizabeth Akesson
Patricia Stewart
Siân Spacey

Acknowledgments

We continue to be grateful to the many colleagues and students who contributed to the first edition of *Cranial Nerves*. From the University of Toronto, they include Dr. E. G. (Mike) Bertram, Department of Anatomy; Professor Stephen Gilbert, Department of Art as Applied to Medicine; Dr. Peter Carlen, Addiction Research Foundation Clinical Institute, Playfair Neuroscience Institute, Departments of Medicine (Neurology) and Physiology; Mr. Ted Davis, first-year medical student; Mr. Steve Toussaint (deceased), Chief Technician, Department of Anatomy; and Ms. Pam Topham, Anatomy Department Secretary. Our colleagues also include, from the University of Manitoba, Dr. C. R. Braekevelt and Dr. J. S. Thliveris from the Department of Anatomy.

In this second edition, we would like to acknowledge the many colleagues who have contributed to our new work. From the University of Toronto, they include Dr. Ray Buncic, Ophthalmologist-in-Chief, Hospital for Sick Children; Ms. Leslie MacKeen, Dr. Buncic's Surgical Assistant; Dr. Dianne Broussard, Department of Physiology; Dr. R. V. Harrison, Department of Otolaryngology, Hospital for Sick Children; Dr. Marika Hohol, Department of Neurology; and Profs. Jodie Jenkinson (the creator of the Cranial Nerves Examination on CD-ROM), Nick Woolridge, and David Mazierski, Division of Biomedical Communications, Department of Surgery. From the University of British Columbia, they are Dr. Joanne Weinberg, Department of Anatomy; Dr. Wayne Vogl, Department of Anatomy; Dr. Tony Pearson, Department of Physiology; and Dr. Roger Nugent, Vancouver General Hospital. Finally, from the University of Manitoba, we thank Dr. C. R. Braekevelt, Department of Anatomy, who is now retired and living in Perth, Australia.

We are especially grateful to our student readers who ensured that our writing was appropriate for our target audience. From the University of Toronto, they are Ms. Melissa Bayne and Mr. Simon McVaugh-Smock, Department of Speech and Language Pathology, and Ms. Allison Guy, Faculty of Arts and Science; and from the University of British Columbia, Ms. Maria Glavas, Department of Anatomy.

We would also like to acknowledge the following medical illustrators: Ms. Andrée Jenks for providing the animations on CD-ROM and Mr. Chesley Sheppard for being the model in the "Cranial Nerves Examination" section on CD-ROM.

Also, to the physicians who provided medical images to supplement our case histories, we would like to extend a special thanks: Dr. Robert Nugent, Vancouver General Hospital, University of British Columbia (Figure I–1); Dr. Ray Buncic (noted above) (Figures II–2 and II–16); Dr. David Mikulis, Department of Medical Imaging, University of Toronto (Figure V–15); and Dr. D. S. Butcher, William Osler Health Centre, Brampton, Ontario (Figure VIII–9).

We are pleased that this second edition of *Cranial Nerves* is again published by BC Decker Inc and would like to take this opportunity to thank the president, Mr. Brian Decker, for his continued support in the development of this textbook. We also extend a special thank you to our colleagues at BC Decker Inc for their advice and thorough editing of this production.

Content

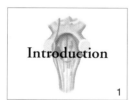
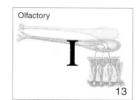
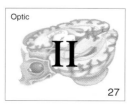
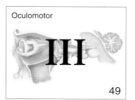
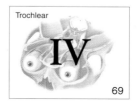
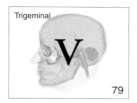
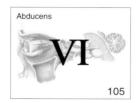
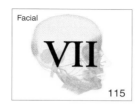
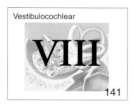
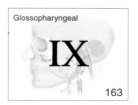
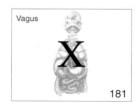
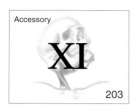
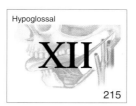
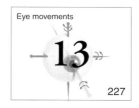

User's Guide

The second edition of *Cranial Nerves* has a number of unique features that enhance the text by providing the reader with additional information and instruction. The visual markers illustrated below can be found throughout the book and alert the reader to these expanded elements.

 This icon indicates that the graphic is animated on the CD-ROM.

TEXT SET IN GRAY BOXES

This text provides additional relevant information that is not essential for understanding the basics of cranial nerve anatomy and function but may be of interest to readers.

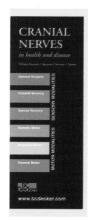

BOOKMARK

The flap on the back cover serves as both a bookmark and a legend. It summarizes a unique feature of this book—the color-coded nerve modalities. They involve three sensory tracts (general, visceral, and special) and three motor tracts, (somatic, branchial, and visceral).

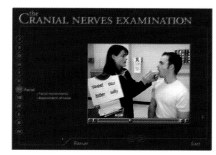

CD-ROM

The accompanying dual-platform CD-ROM features the complete text of the book and high resolution graphics, in fully searchable PDF files, that can be magnified for greater detail. Several of these graphics are animated to show cellular processes associated with cranial nerves. The CD also features the program "Cranial Nerves Examination," which takes you step by step through the testing process.

Cranial Nerves | Introduction

*the
cranial nerves
provide
sensory and motor
innervation
for the
head and neck*

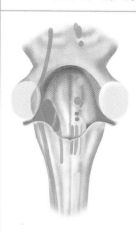

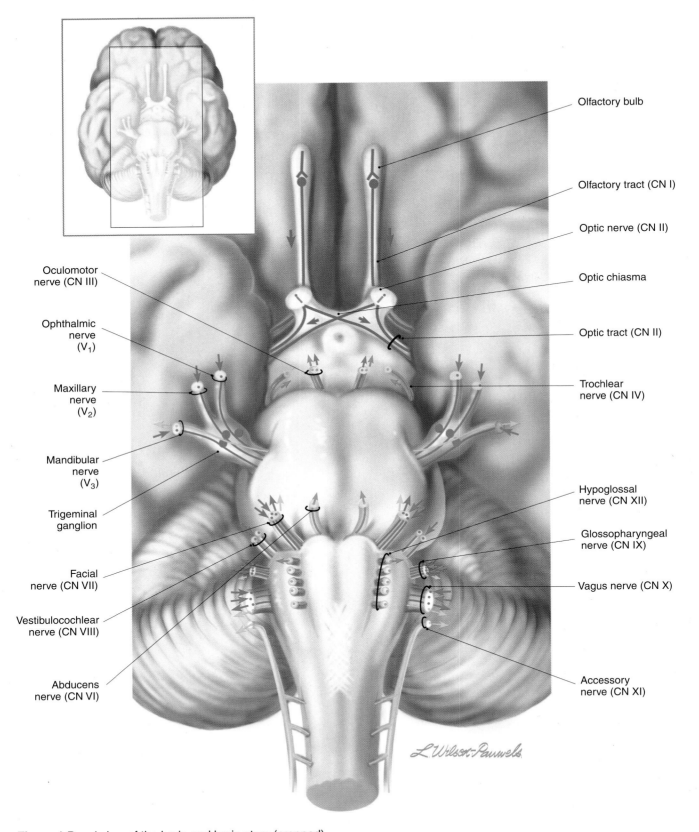

Olfactory bulb

Olfactory tract (CN I)

Optic nerve (CN II)

Optic chiasma

Optic tract (CN II)

Trochlear nerve (CN IV)

Hypoglossal nerve (CN XII)

Glossopharyngeal nerve (CN IX)

Vagus nerve (CN X)

Accessory nerve (CN XI)

Oculomotor nerve (CN III)

Ophthalmic nerve (V$_1$)

Maxillary nerve (V$_2$)

Mandibular nerve (V$_3$)

Trigeminal ganglion

Facial nerve (CN VII)

Vestibulocochlear nerve (CN VIII)

Abducens nerve (CN VI)

L. Wilson-Pauwels

Figure 1 Basal view of the brain and brain stem (cropped).

Introduction

COMPONENTS OF CRANIAL NERVES

The cranial nerves provide sensory and motor innervation for the head and neck including general and special sensory and voluntary and involuntary muscle control. Because they emerge from the cranium, they are called *cranial* nerves as opposed to spinal nerves that emerge from the spinal column.

The cranial nerves function as modified spinal nerves. As a group, they have both sensory and motor* components; however, individual nerves may be purely sensory, purely motor, or mixed (both motor and sensory).

The cranial nerves carry *six distinct modalities*—three sensory and three motor (Figure 1 and Tables 1 and 2). These modalities are

- **general sensory,** which perceives touch, pain, temperature, pressure, vibration, and proprioceptive sensation;
- **visceral sensory,** which perceives sensory input, except pain, from the viscera;
- **special sensory,** which perceives smell, vision, taste, hearing, and balance;
- **somatic motor,** which innervates the muscles that develop from the somites;
- **branchial motor,** which innervates the muscles that develop from the branchial arches; and
- **visceral motor,** which innervates the viscera, including glands and all smooth muscle.

In this book each modality has been assigned a different color, and the color scheme is adhered to throughout. Figure 1 provides an overview of the base of the brain and brain stem with the cranial nerves in situ. Tables 1 and 2 provide a summary of the cranial nerves, their modalities, and their functions.

---

*In this text we have chosen to use the words "sensory" and "motor" rather than the terms "afferent" and "efferent," which are internationally recognized and detailed in *Terminologica Anatomica*. In written work, the use of afferent and efferent appeals to scholars because it avoids the difficulties in defining motor and sensory by describing only the direction of the impulse. In lectures, however, afferent and efferent sound so much alike that the students find them difficult to distinguish, and we have found their use to be confusing.

Table 1 Cranial Nerves, Modalities, and Functions

Nerve	Sensory Modalities			Motor Modalities			Function
	General	Visceral	Special	Somatic	Branchial	Visceral	(For more detail see appropriate chapter)
Olfactory CN I			✔				Special sensory for smell
Optic CN II			✔				Special sensory for vision
Oculomotor CN III				✔		✔	Somatic motor to all extraocular muscles except superior oblique and lateral rectus muscles Parasympathetic motor supply to ciliary and constrictor pupillae muscles
Trochlear CN IV				✔			Somatic motor to superior oblique muscle
Trigeminal CN V	✔				✔		General sensory from face, anterior scalp, eyes, sinuses, nasal and oral cavities, anterior two-thirds of tongue, meninges of anterior and middle cranial fossae, and external tympanic membrane Branchial motor to muscles of mastication, tensores tympani and veli palatini, and mylohyoid and anterior belly of digastric muscles
Abducens CN VI				✔			Somatic motor to lateral rectus muscle
Facial CN VII	✔		✔		✔	✔	General sensory from skin of choncha of auricle, behind the external ear, and external tympanic membrane Special sensory for taste from anterior two-thirds of tongue Branchial motor to muscles of facial expression Parasympathetic to lacrimal glands, submandibular and sublingual glands, and oral and nasal mucosa
Vestibular division CN VIII Cochlear division CN VIII			✔ ✔				Special sensory for balance Special sensory for hearing
Glossopharyngeal CN IX	✔	✔	✔		✔	✔	General sensory from posterior one-third of tongue, tonsil, skin of external ear, internal surface of tympanic membrane, and pharnyx Visceral sensory from the carotid body and sinus Special sensory for taste from posterior one-third of tongue Branchial motor to stylopharyngeus muscle Parasympathetic to parotid gland and blood vessels in carotid body
Vagus CN X	✔	✔			✔	✔	General sensory from a small area around the external ear, posterior meninges, external tympanic membrane, and larynx Visceral sensory from pharynx, larynx, and thoracic and abdominal viscera including aortic bodies Branchial motor to pharyngeal (including palatoglossus) and laryngeal muscles Parasympathetic supply to smooth muscles and glands of the pharynx, larynx, and thoracic and abdominal viscera, and cardiac muscle
Accessory CN XI					✔		Branchial motor to sternomastoid and trapezius muscles
Hypoglossal CN XII				✔			Somatic motor to intrinsic and extrinsic muscles of the tongue except palatoglossus

Table 2 Modalities, Cranial Nerves, Nuclei, and Functions

Modality	Nerve	Nucleus	Function
General sensory	CN V	Trigeminal	Face, anterior scalp, eyes, sinuses, nasal and oral cavities, anterior two-thirds of tongue, meninges of anterior and middle cranial fossae, and external tympanic membrane
	CN VII	Trigeminal	Skin of choncha of auricle, behind the external ear, and external tympanic membrane
	CN IX	Trigeminal	Posterior one-third of tongue, skin of external ear, internal surface of tympanic membrane, the tonsil, and pharynx
	CN X	Trigeminal	Small area around external ear, external tympanic membrane, posterior meninges, and larynx
Visceral sensory	CN IX	Solitarius*	Carotid body and sinus
	CN X	Solitarius*	Pharynx, larynx, and thoracic and abdominal viscera including aortic bodies
Special sensory†	CN I	Mitral cells of olfactory bulb	Smell
	CN II	Ganglion cells of retina	Vision
	CN VII	Gustatory‡	Taste—anterior two-thirds of tongue
	CN VIII	Vestibular	Balance
	CN VIII	Cochlear	Hearing
	CN IX	Gustatory‡	Taste—posterior one-third of tongue
Somatic motor	CN III	Oculomotor	All extraocular eye muscles except superior oblique and lateral rectus
	CN IV	Trochlear	Superior oblique muscle
	CN VI	Abducens	Lateral rectus muscle
	CN XII	Hypoglossal	Intrinsic and extrinsic tongue muscles except palatoglossus
Branchial motor	CN V	Masticator	Muscles of mastication, tensores tympani and veli palatini, and mylohyoid and anterior belly of digastric muscles
	CN VII	Facial	Muscles of facial expression
	CN IX	Ambiguus	Stylopharyngeus muscle
	CN X	Ambiguus	Muscles of pharynx, including palatoglossus, and larynx
	CN XI	Accessory§	Sternomastoid and trapezius muscles
Visceral motor (parasympathetic)	CN III	Edinger-Westphal	Ciliary and constrictor pupillae muscles
	CN VII	Superior salivatory	Lacrimal glands, submandibular and sublingual glands, and oral and nasal mucosa
	CN IX	Inferior salivatory	Parotid gland, blood vessels in carotid body
	CN X	Dorsal vagal	Smooth muscles and glands of the pharynx, larynx, and thoracic and abdominal viscera
	CN X	Ambiguus	Cardiac muscle

*More properly known as the nucleus of the tractus solitarius.
†Special sensory nuclei are defined as the cell bodies of the secondary sensory neurons.
‡The gustatory nucleus is the rostral portion of the nucleus of the tractus solitarius.
§In this text we will not follow the convention of identifying the caudal fibers of cranial nerve X that run briefly with cranial nerve XI as the "cranial root of XI" (see Chapter X for further discussion).

CRANIAL NERVE SENSORY (AFFERENT) PATHWAYS

Sensory pathways are composed of three major neurons: the primary, secondary, and tertiary (Figure 2).

1. The **primary neuron** cell bodies are usually located outside the central nervous system (CNS) in sensory ganglia. They are homologous with the dorsal root ganglia of the spinal cord but are usually smaller and are frequently overlooked.

2. The **secondary neuron** cell bodies are located in the dorsal gray matter of the brain stem, and their axons usually cross the midline to project to the thalamus. The cell bodies that reside in the brain stem form the sensory group of cranial nerve nuclei.

3. The **tertiary neuron** cell bodies are located in the thalamus, and their axons project to the sensory cortex.

The sensory component of the cranial nerves, except for nerves I and II, consists of the axons of the primary sensory neurons. Cranial nerves I and II are special cases that will be explained in the appropriate chapters. The afferent fibers of the primary sensory neurons enter the brain stem and terminate on the secondary sensory neurons, which form the sensory nuclei.

Since there are several modalities carried by sensory neurons, and since these modalities tend to follow different pathways in the brain stem, the loss experienced when sensory neurons are damaged depends, to a large extent, on the location of the lesion.

- Lesions in a peripheral nerve result in the loss of all sensation carried by that nerve from its field of distribution.
- Sensory abnormalities resulting from lesions in the central nervous system depend on which sensory pathways are affected. For example, a lesion in the descending portion of the trigeminal nucleus results in loss of pain and temperature sensation on the affected side of the face but in little loss of discriminative touch, which is perceived in the middle and upper part of the same nucleus (see Chapter V, Figure V–10).
- Damage to the thalamus results in a patchy hemianesthesia (numbness) and hemianalgesia (insensitivity to pain) on the contralateral (opposite) side of the body. There is often additional spontaneous pain of an unpleasant, disturbing nature on the partially anesthetized side.

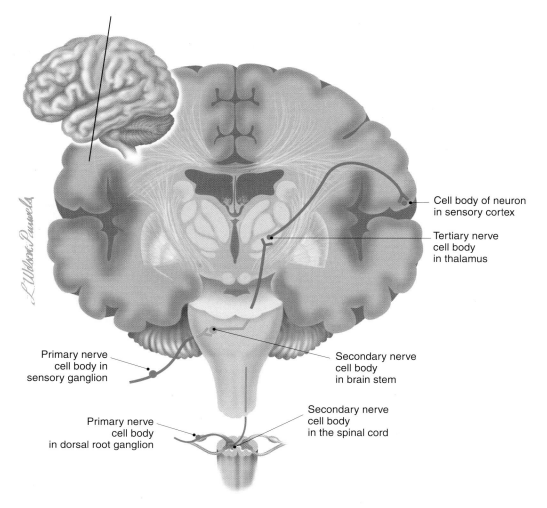

Figure 2 Typical sensory pathway.

CRANIAL NERVE MOTOR (EFFERENT) PATHWAYS

Motor pathways (somatic and branchial) are composed of two major neurons: the upper motor neuron and the lower motor neuron (Figure 3).

1. The **upper motor neuron** is usually located in the cerebral cortex. Its axon projects caudally through the corticobulbar tract* to contact the lower motor neuron. Most, but not all, of the motor pathways that terminate in the brain stem project bilaterally to contact lower motor neurons on both sides of the midline.

*The term "corticobulbar" describes upper motor neuron axons originating in the cortex and terminating in nuclei in the brain stem (bulb).

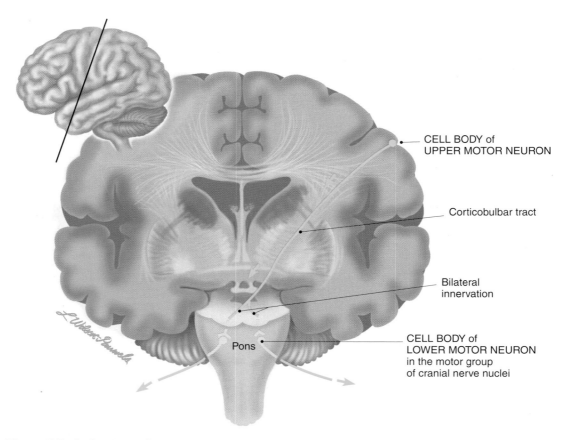

CELL BODY of
UPPER MOTOR NEURON

Corticobulbar tract

Bilateral
innervation

CELL BODY of
LOWER MOTOR NEURON
in the motor group
of cranial nerve nuclei

Pons

Figure 3 Typical motor pathway.

Damage to any part of the upper motor neuron results in an upper motor neuron lesion (UMNL). The symptoms of an upper motor neuron lesion include

- paresis (weakness) or paralysis when voluntary movement is attempted;
- increased muscle tone ("spasticity"); and
- exaggerated tendon reflexes.

Wasting of the muscles does not occur unless the paralysis is present for some time, at which point some degree of disuse atrophy appears. These symptoms do not occur in those parts of the body that are bilaterally represented in the cortex. In the head and neck, all the muscles are bilaterally represented except the sternomastoid, trapezius, and those of the lower half of the face and tongue.

2. The **lower motor neuron** is located in the brain stem (Figure 4) or upper cervical spinal cord. The cell bodies form the motor cranial nerve nuclei. Axons that leave these nuclei make up the motor component of the cranial nerves.

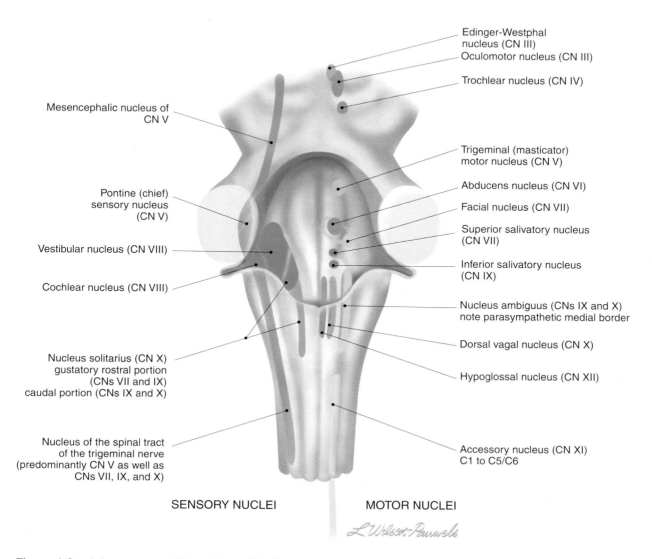

Edinger-Westphal
nucleus (CN III)

Oculomotor nucleus (CN III)

Trochlear nucleus (CN IV)

Mesencephalic nucleus of
CN V

Trigeminal (masticator)
motor nucleus (CN V)

Pontine (chief)
sensory nucleus
(CN V)

Abducens nucleus (CN VI)

Facial nucleus (CN VII)

Superior salivatory nucleus
(CN VII)

Vestibular nucleus (CN VIII)

Inferior salivatory nucleus
(CN IX)

Cochlear nucleus (CN VIII)

Nucleus ambiguus (CNs IX and X)
note parasympathetic medial border

Dorsal vagal nucleus (CN X)

Nucleus solitarius (CN X)
gustatory rostral portion
(CNs VII and IX)
caudal portion (CNs IX and X)

Hypoglossal nucleus (CN XII)

Nucleus of the spinal tract
of the trigeminal nerve
(predominantly CN V as well as
CNs VII, IX, and X)

Accessory nucleus (CN XI)
C1 to C5/C6

SENSORY NUCLEI   MOTOR NUCLEI

L. Wilson-Pauwels

Figure 4 Cranial nerve nuclei (dorsal view of brain stem).

Damage to any part of the lower motor neuron results in a lower motor neuron lesion (LMNL). The symptoms of a lower motor neuron lesion include

- paresis (weakness) or, if all the motor neurons to a particular muscle group are affected, complete paralysis;
- loss of muscle tone ("flaccidity");
- loss of tendon reflexes;
- rapid atrophy of the affected muscles; and
- fasciculation (random twitching of small muscle groups).

CRANIAL NERVES VISCERAL MOTOR (PARASYMPATHETIC EFFERENT) PATHWAYS

The visceral motor (parasympathetic) pathway differs from the somatic/branchial motor pathways in that it is a three-neuron chain. Its target includes smooth and cardiac muscle and secretory cells (Figure 5).

- **First-order neurons** in higher centers project to parasympathetic nuclei in the brain stem.

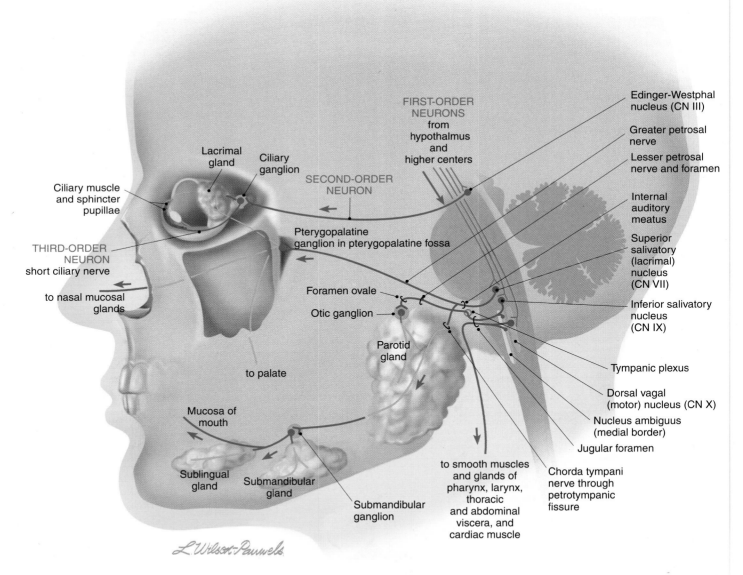

Figure 5 Visceral motor (parasympathetic) component of the head and neck.

- **Second-order neurons** from the nuclei project via cranial nerves III, VII, IX, and X to ganglia located outside the central nervous system.
- **Third-order neurons** from these ganglia travel with peripheral branches of cranial nerves III, VII , IX, and X to reach their targets in the head, thorax, and abdomen.

The parasympathetic nuclei are the Edinger-Westphal nucleus, the superior and inferior salivatory nuclei, the dorsal vagal nucleus, and the medial aspect of nucleus ambiguus. They are under the influence of higher centers in the diencephalon and brain stem, namely the hypothalamus, olfactory system, and autonomic centers in the reticular formation.

Visceral motor axons from the Edinger-Westphal nucleus in the midbrain, travel in cranial nerve III through the cavernous sinus and superior orbital fissure to terminate in the ciliary ganglion near the apex of the orbit. Postganglionic axons leave the ganglion as the short ciliary nerves to end in the ciliary muscle that controls the shape of the lens in visual accommodation and in the sphincter pupillae to constrict the pupil (see Chapter III).

The facial nerve (cranial nerve VII) is associated with two parasympathetic ganglia. Visceral motor axons from the superior salivatory nucleus in the brain stem travel through the internal auditory meatus into the facial canal where they divide into two bundles. One, the greater petrosal nerve, reaches the pterygopalatine ganglion in the pterygopalatine fossa. Postganglionic fibers pass to the mucosal glands of the nose and palate and to the lacrimal glands. The second bundle travels in the chorda tympani nerve, which joins the lingual nerve (V_2) and synapses in the submandibular ganglion suspended from the lingual nerve. From the ganglion, postsynaptic fibers travel to the submandibular and sublingual glands and the mucosa of the mouth to stimulate secretion (see Chapter VII).

The glossopharyngeal nerve (cranial nerve IX) carries axons originating in the inferior salivatory nucleus. These axons project through the tympanic plexus, the lesser petrosal foramen, and the foramen ovale to synapse in the otic ganglion. Postganglionic neurons within the ganglion innervate secretory cells and smooth muscle within the parotid gland (see Chapter IX).

Visceral motor axons in the vagus nerve (cranial nerve X) originate in the dorsal vagal (motor) nucleus and in the medial aspect of the nucleus ambiguus. They end on small ganglia (pulmonary, cardiac, and enteric ganglia) within the walls of the viscera. Postganglionic neurons within the ganglia innervate secretory cells and smooth muscle cells within the viscera (see Chapter X).

I Olfactory Nerve

*carries the
special sense
of smell*

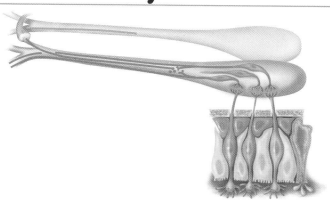

I Olfactory Nerve

CASE HISTORY

Anne, a medical student, was riding to classes when she was knocked off her bicycle at an intersection. She hit the back of her head, suffered a brief loss of consciousness, and was subsequently taken to the hospital. On examination, she was found to have some superficial bruising on her body and was tender over the back (occiput) of her skull. Otherwise she appeared alert and well. A skull radiograph revealed a fracture starting at the base of her skull extending through the cribriform plate. Anne was admitted to the hospital for observation overnight.

In the morning, Anne complained that she could not smell anything and, in fact, she could not taste her breakfast. In addition, she had noticed a constant clear discharge from her nose. A computed tomography (CT) scan confirmed the basal skull fracture, and no other abnormalities were seen (Figure I–1). More complete testing of her cranial nerve function revealed that her sense of smell was absent. However, direct testing of her taste (cranial nerves VII and IX) continued to be normal. During the next 24 hours, the nasal discharge subsided and eventually Anne was discharged from the hospital.

Five years later, Anne's sense of smell still has not recovered. Her appreciation of food has changed greatly and, although the doctors tell her that her taste pathways are intact, food continues to be tasteless.

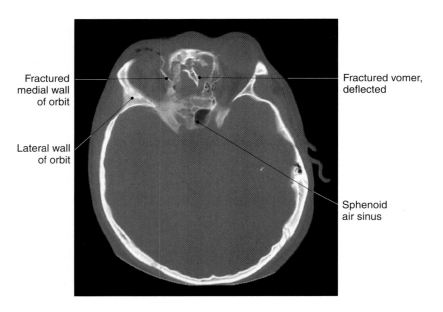

Fractured medial wall of orbit

Lateral wall of orbit

Fractured vomer, deflected

Sphenoid air sinus

Figure I–1 Computed tomography (CT) scan through the vomer showing fractures of the vomer, sphenoid, and medial wall of the orbit. Because the scan is taken in the axial plane, the same plane as the cribriform plate, the fracture of the cribriform plate is not visualized in this image. (Courtesy of Dr. Robert Nugent.)

OLFACTORY NERVE ANATOMY

The olfactory nerve* functions in the special sense of olfaction or smell, hence its name (Table I–1). The structures in the central nervous system (CNS) that are involved in olfaction are collectively called the rhinencephalon, or "nose" brain. The olfactory system is remarkable in that

- peripheral processes of the primary sensory neurons in the olfactory epithelium (Figure I–2) act as sensory receptors (unlike the other special sensory nerves that have separate receptors);
- primary afferent neurons undergo continuous replacement throughout life;

Table I–1 Nerve Fiber Modality and Function of the Olfactory Nerve

Nerve Fiber Modality	Function
Special sensory (afferent)	Sensation of olfaction or smell

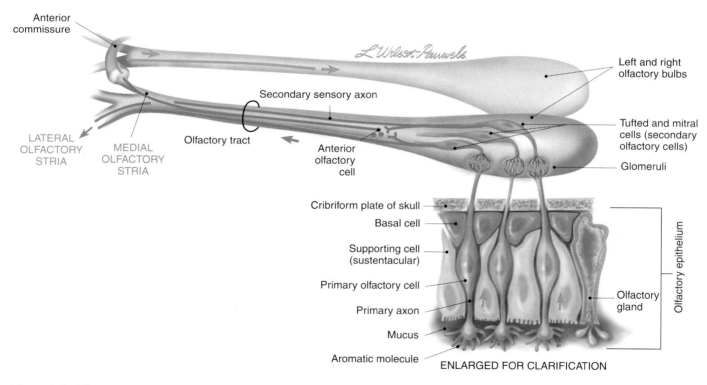

Figure I–2 Olfactory epilthelium, bulb, and tracts.

*The primary olfactory nerve cell bodies send central processes to synapse on secondary olfactory cells in the olfactory bulb. Secondary sensory axons then form the olfactory tract. Traditionally, however, the bulb and tract are known as the olfactory "nerve."

- primary afferent neurons synapse with secondary neurons in the olfactory bulb (an outgrowth of cortex) without synapsing first in the thalamus (as do all other sensory neurons); and
- pathways to the cortical areas involved in olfaction are entirely ipsilateral.

The olfactory system is made up of the olfactory epithelium, bulbs, and tracts, together with olfactory areas in the brain and their communications with other brain centers.

Olfactory Epithelium

The olfactory epithelium (see Figure I–2) is located in the roof of the nasal cavity and extends onto the superior nasal conchae and the nasal septum. The epithelium is kept moist by olfactory glandular secretions, and it is in this moisture that inhaled scents (aromatic molecules) are dissolved. The epithelium comprises three cell types.

1. **Olfactory neurons** are bipolar neurons whose peripheral processes (dendrites) extend to the epithelial surface where they expand into an olfactory knob with cilia, which contain the molecular receptor sites. These primary sensory neurons transmit sensation via central processes, which assemble into twenty or more bundles or filaments that traverse the cribriform plate of the ethmoid bone to synapse on the secondary sensory neurons in the olfactory bulb.

2. **Sustentacular cells** (supporting cells) are intermingled with the sensory cells and are similar to glia.

3. **Basal cells** lie on the basement membrane and are the source of new receptor cells. This is the only area of the central nervous system where cells are continuously regenerated throughout life. Regeneration occurs over a period of about 60 days.

Olfactory Bulb

The olfactory bulb is the rostral enlargement of the olfactory tract. The olfactory bulbs and tracts are parts of the brain that evaginated from the telencephalon in early development. The olfactory bulb contains the cell bodies of the secondary sensory neurons involved in the relay of olfactory sensation to the brain. The olfactory bulb contains spherical structures called glomeruli in which contact between the primary olfactory neurons and mitral cells and tufted cells (secondary olfactory neurons) takes place. Starting at the cribriform plate, the bulb is arranged in five layers (Figure I–3).

1. The nerve fiber layer (olfactory axons) is the most superficial layer, which contains the axons of primary olfactory neurons in the nasal mucosa.

2. The glomerular layer contains spherical glomeruli in which considerable convergence takes place between the axons of primary olfactory neurons and the

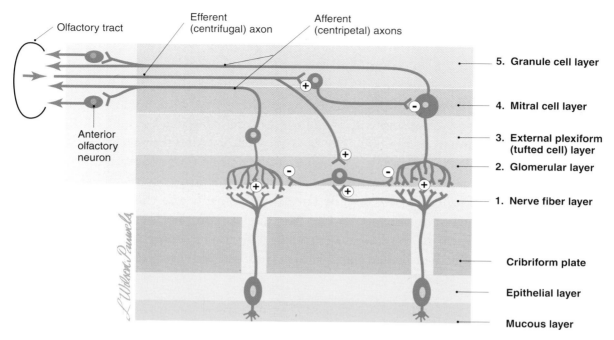

Figure I–3 Olfactory pathway from olfactory epithelium to the olfactory tract. Numbers 1 to 5 represent the layers of the olfactory bulb. The olfactory tract includes afferent (second order) axons of tufted and mitral cells; neurons of the anterior olfactory nucleus; and efferent axons from the olfactory cortex and from the contralateral olfactory nucleus.

dendrites of tufted and mitral cells, as well as input from interneurons and centrifugal efferents from the central nervous system.

3. The external plexiform layer contains mainly the bodies of tufted cells.

4. The mitral cell layer is a single layer of large mitral cell bodies.

5. The granule cell layer contains granule cells (inhibitory interneurons) and myelinated axons of secondary neurons.

Within the layers are two major cell types. These are:

1. Mitral cells whose dendrites extend into the glomeruli where they are contacted by the axons of primary sensory neurons and by interneurons. After giving off collaterals to the anterior olfactory nucleus, the mitral cell axons project mainly to the lateral (primary) olfactory area.

2. Tufted cells whose dendrites extend into the glomeruli where they also make contact with the axons of primary olfactory neurons. Their axons project to the anterior olfactory nucleus and to the lateral and intermediate areas.

The tufted and mitral cells are functionally similar and together constitute the afferent neurons from the olfactory bulb to the CNS. Periglomerular interneurons interact between glomeruli. There is a high incidence of convergence within the glomerular layer as well as input from the central nervous system.

Olfactory Bulb Projections

From the olfactory bulb, the postsynaptic fibers of these sensory neurons form the olfactory tract and trigone (an expansion of the olfactory tract just rostral to the anterior perforated substance of the brain). These fibers divide in front of the anterior perforated substance into lateral and medial olfactory striae to convey impulses to olfactory areas for the conscious appreciation of smell (Figures I–4 and I–5).

Most of the axons from the olfactory tract pass via the lateral olfactory stria to the primary (lateral) olfactory area. The olfactory area consists of the cortices of the uncus and entorhinal area (anterior part of the parahippocampal gyrus), the limen insula (the point of junction between the cortex of the insula and the cortex of the frontal lobe), and part of the amygdaloid body (a nuclear complex located above the tip of the inferior horn of the lateral ventricle). The uncus, entorhinal area, and limen insulae are collectively called the pyriform (pear shaped) area (see Figure I–5).

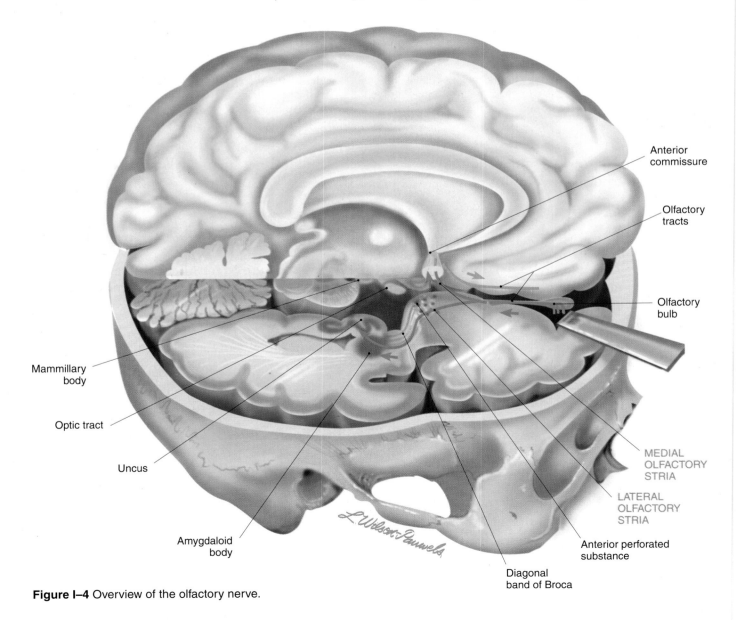

Figure I–4 Overview of the olfactory nerve.

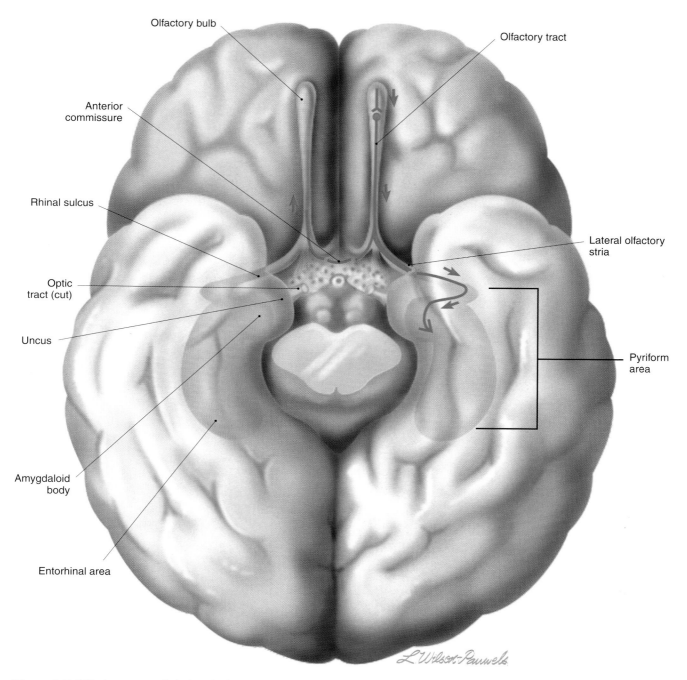

Olfactory bulb

Olfactory tract

Anterior
commissure

Rhinal sulcus

Lateral olfactory
stria

Optic
tract (cut)

Uncus

Pyriform
area

Amygdaloid
body

Entorhinal area

L. Wilson-Pauwels

Figure I–5 Olfactory areas (inferior view).

Unlike other sensory modalities whose axons synapse in the thalamus before terminating in the cortex, olfactory secondary neurons project directly to the olfactory
cortex from the olfactory bulb and then have direct connections to the limbic area.
The limbic area plays a role in forming and consolidating memories. It is this close
association with the limbic region that explains why certain smells are so evoca-
tive of memory and emotion.

From the primary olfactory areas, projections go to the olfactory association area in the entorhinal cortex (Brodmann's area 28), the hypothalamus, and to the dorsal medial nucleus of the thalamus from which afferent neurons project to the orbitofrontal cortex for the conscious appreciation of smell.

Some collateral branches of the axons of the secondary sensory neurons terminate in a small group of cells called the anterior olfactory nucleus, which is a collection of nerve cell bodies located along the olfactory tract. Postsynaptic fibers from this nucleus travel either with the central processes of the mitral and tufted cells or travel in the medial olfactory stria to enter the anterior commissure whereby they reach the contralateral olfactory bulb (see Figure I–2). Their influence on the contralateral olfactory bulb is mainly inhibitory. This serves to enhance the more active bulb and provide directional cues to the source of the olfactory stimulation.

The olfactory system shares the entorhinal cortex with the limbic system, which has extensive connections with the septal area (formerly designated the medial olfactory area) of the frontal cortex and the hypothalamus with its autonomic centers.

Major Projections of the Olfactory Cortical Areas

The olfactory system is a complex communications network. Cells of the olfactory cortex have reciprocal connections with other regions in the olfactory cortex and outside the cortical areas. They contribute to fibers reaching the autonomic centers for visceral responses, such as salivation in response to pleasant cooking odors or nausea in response to unpleasant odors. The principal pathways (Figure I–6) are

- the medial forebrain bundle (information from all olfactory areas to the hypothalamus and brain stem reticular formation);
- the stria medullaris thalami (olfactory stimuli from the various olfactory areas to the habenular nucleus [epithalamus]);
- the stria terminalis (information from the amygdala to the anterior hypothalamus and the preoptic area);
- the dorsal longitudinal fasciculus (information from the hypothalamus to the brain stem and spinal cord); and
- the habenular nucleus and the hypothalamus project to the brain stem reticular formation and the cranial nerve nuclei, which are responsible for visceral responses: for example, the superior and inferior salivatory nuclei and the dorsal vagal nucleus (acceleration of peristalsis in the intestinal tract and increased gastric secretion).

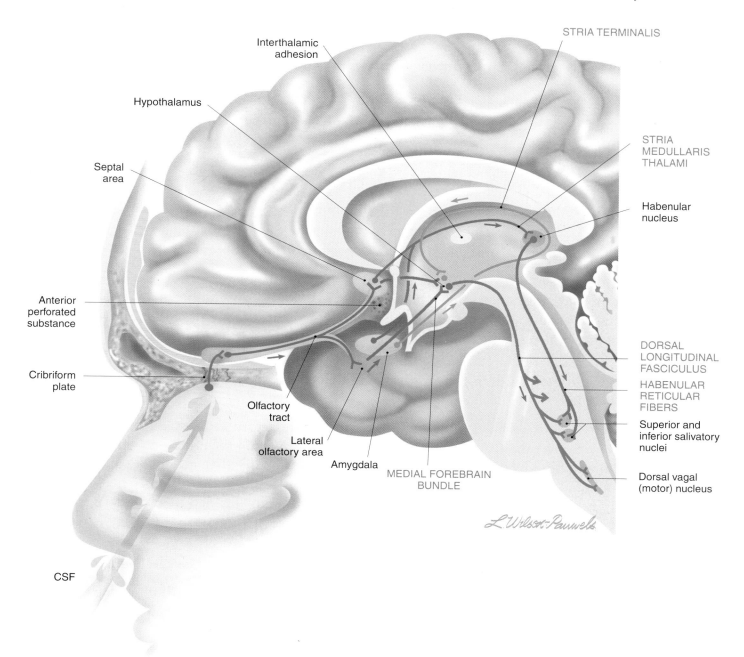

STRIA TERMINALIS

Interthalamic
adhesion

STRIA
MEDULLARIS
THALAMI

Hypothalamus

Habenular
nucleus

Septal
area

Anterior
perforated
substance

DORSAL
LONGITUDINAL
FASCICULUS

HABENULAR
RETICULAR
FIBERS

Cribriform
plate

Superior and
inferior salivatory
nuclei

Olfactory
tract

Dorsal vagal
(motor) nucleus

Lateral
olfactory area

Amygdala

MEDIAL FOREBRAIN
BUNDLE

L. Wilson-Pauwels

CSF

Figure I–6 Major olfactory pathways. CSF = cerebrospinal fluid.

CASE HISTORY GUIDING QUESTIONS

1. What is anosmia, and why has Anne developed this problem?

2. How do molecules in the air give rise to electrical signals in olfactory neurons?

3. How is the sense of smell carried from the nasal mucosa to the cerebrum?

4. Where along the olfactory pathway can pathology occur?

5. What is the nasal discharge from Anne's nose?

6. Why is the patient's sense of taste diminished?

1. What is anosmia, and why has Anne developed this problem?

Anosmia is loss of the sense of smell. When Anne fell off her bicycle, she hit the back of her head on the concrete. The blow resulted in an anteroposterior movement of the brain within the cranium. Olfactory axons (filaments) were sheared off at the cribriform plate resulting in disruption of the olfactory pathway.

2. How do molecules in the air give rise to electrical signals in olfactory neurons?

Odorants, that is, airborne molecules that stimulate olfactory neurons, dissolve in the mucous layer that covers the olfactory epithelium. Within the mucus they bind to odorant binding proteins, small water soluble proteins that act to dissolve hydrophobic odorants, and diffuse into the ciliary processes of the olfactory neurons. There they bind to olfactory receptors, which are embedded in the ciliary membrane (Figure I–7).

3. How is the sense of smell carried from the nasal mucosa to the cerebrum?

Primary sensory neurons in the nasal mucosa project to the olfactory bulb where they synapse with second-order neurons. The secondary olfactory cells project centrally via the (a) lateral olfactory stria to the primary olfactory area in the temporal lobe of the brain, and (b) medial olfactory stria to the septal area of the brain (see Figure I–4).

4. Where along the olfactory pathway can pathology occur?

Pathology can occur anywhere along the olfactory pathway. However, it is easiest to consider in terms of the receptor, the primary axon (filament), and the central pathway.

- *The Receptor*

    Temporary loss of smell results, most commonly, from swelling and congestion of the nasal mucosa due to the common cold or allergic rhinitis, which prevents

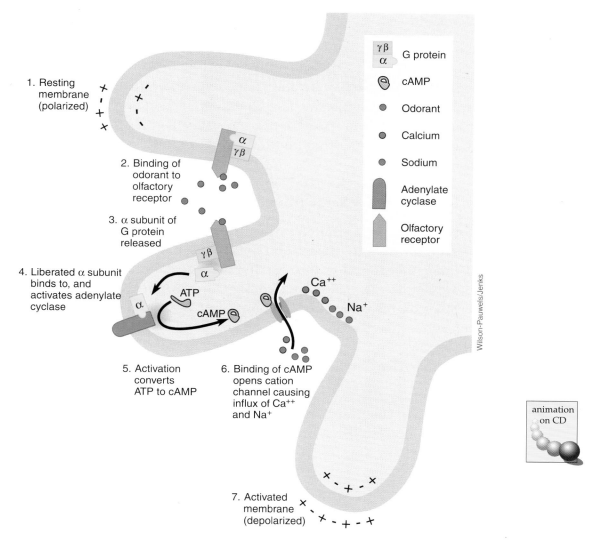

1. Resting membrane (polarized)

2. Binding of odorant to olfactory receptor

3. α subunit of G protein released

4. Liberated α subunit binds to, and activates adenylate cyclase

5. Activation converts ATP to cAMP

6. Binding of cAMP opens cation channel causing influx of Ca++ and Na+

7. Activated membrane (depolarized)

γβ / α   G protein

cAMP

Odorant

Calcium

Sodium

Adenylate cyclase

Olfactory receptor

Wilson-Pauwels/Jenks

animation on CD

Figure I–7 Activation (depolarization) of an olfactory neuron. ATP = adenosine triphosphate; cAMP = cyclic adenosine monophosphate.

olfactory stimuli (odorants) from reaching the receptor cells. The receptors themselves can be damaged by chronic smoking and viral infections such as herpes simplex, influenza, and hepatitis. In rare instances, tumors of the olfactory epithelium can arise and are referred to as esthesioneuroepitheliomas.

- *The Primary Axon (Filament)*

The receptor cells (primary olfactory neurons) transmit their information via axons (processes or filaments) that traverse the cribriform plate of the ethmoid bone to synapse on the secondary sensory neurons in the olfactory bulb. A blow to the head may cause a shift of the brain resulting in shearing of the delicate filaments as they pass through the bony cribriform plate. This may result in permanent unilateral or bilateral anosmia and is frequently seen with fractures through the cribriform plate.

- *The Central Pathway*

The central olfactory pathway includes the olfactory bulb, the olfactory tract, and its central projections. The olfactory bulb may become contused or lacerated from head injury. The location of the bulbs and tracts makes them susceptible to compression from olfactory groove meningiomas, aneurysms of the anterior cerebral artery or the anterior communicating artery, and infiltrating tumors of the frontal lobe. Such compression injuries may result in either unilateral or bilateral loss of smell.

5. What is the nasal discharge from Anne's nose?

Anne's closed head injury resulted in a fracture of the cribriform plate with a subsequent tearing of the dura mater and arachnoid mater. The discharge was cerebrospinal fluid (CSF) leaking through the dural tear into the nasopharynx. The leakage of CSF from the nose is referred to as CSF rhinorrhea (see Figure I–6).

The CSF discharge is clear and does not cause excoriation within or outside the nose. The patient describes it as salty tasting.

6. Why is the patient's sense of taste diminished?

Ageusia is loss of the sense of taste (see Chapters VII and IX). Perception of flavor is a combination of smell and taste as well as stored memories of the taste of familiar foods. When one contribution to the flavor experience is lost, the overall effect is diminished taste.

CLINICAL TESTING

The olfactory nerve is frequently overlooked in the neurologic examination. However, identification of anosmia is a helpful localizing neurologic finding. The examiner easily can assess the olfactory nerve in the clinical setting by asking the patient to close his eyes while presenting a series of nonirritating, familiar olfactory stimuli such as coffee or chocolate (Figure I–8). The aromatic stimulus should be placed under one nostril while the other nostril is occluded. The patient is asked to sniff the substance and then identify it. The procedure is repeated for the other nostril. If the patient can name or describe the substance, it is assumed that the olfactory tract is intact. Stimuli such as ammonia are unsuitable because they have an irritative effect on the free nerve endings in the nasal mucosa.

There are more elaborate tests such as olfactory evoked potentials that can be used for assessing the olfactory pathway; however, these are primarily research tools and are not used in clinical practice. (See also Cranial Nerves Examination on CD-ROM.)

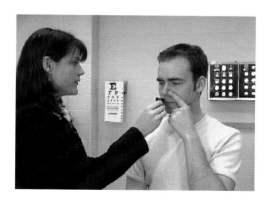

Figure I–8 Identifying olfactory stimuli to test for anosmia.

ADDITIONAL RESOURCES

Bear MF, Connors BW, Paradiso MA. Neuroscience: exploring the brain. Baltimore: Williams & Wilkins; 1996. p. 190–208.

Nakamura T, Gold GH. A cyclic nucleotide-gated conductance in olfactory receptor cilia. Nature 1994;325:442–4.

Sweazey RD. Olfaction and taste. In: Haines DE, editor. Fundamental neuroscience. New York: Churchill Livingstone; 1997. p. 321–3.

II Optic Nerve

*carries the
special sense
of vision*

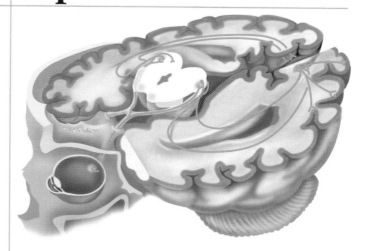

II Optic Nerve

CASE HISTORY

During a photography session, Meredith, a 28-year-old photojournalist, noticed her vision was blurred in her right eye. Initially she thought it was the camera lens, but soon realized the problem was her own eye. Her vision continued to deteriorate over the course of the day. When Meredith awoke the next morning, her vision was markedly blurred and her right eye was now painful, especially when she moved it. Quite alarmed by her symptoms, she went to the emergency department of her local hospital. The attending physician wanted to know about her background and whether she had experienced visual loss or any transient motor or sensory symptoms in the past.

Meredith recalled that she had experienced a minor episode of blurred vision in her left eye about a year previously, but it did not interfere with her activities and got better after one week. She did not see a doctor at the time because she was at the summer cottage and thought that the symptoms were minor.

The doctor took Meredith's history and then examined her. He noticed that although her optic disks appeared normal, her visual acuity was decreased to 20/70 in the right eye, whereas in her left eye it was 20/30. He assessed her color vision and found that she had reduced color discrimination in her right eye as well as decreased contrast sensitivity. When he examined Meredith's visual field, he found that she had a central scotoma (blind area) in her right eye. Both of Meredith's pupils measured 4 mm in diameter. When the doctor shone a bright light into her left eye, both pupils constricted normally; however, when the light was shone in her right eye there was only a slight constriction of the right and left pupils. The doctor then completed the neurologic examination and found that she had no other neurologic abnormalities at this time.

The doctor told Meredith that she had optic neuritis involving her right eye. He told her that her symptoms might progress further over the next couple of days but that they should then start to improve.

ANATOMY OF THE OPTIC NERVE AND VISUAL PATHWAY

The anatomy of the optic nerve is illustrated in Figure II–1. Light enters the eyes and is transformed into electrical signals in the retina. The optic nerve carries these signals to the central nervous system (Table II–1). The optic nerve passes posteromedially from the eye to leave the orbit through the optic canal, which is located in the lesser wing of the sphenoid bone. At the posterior end of the optic canal the optic nerve enters the middle cranial fossa and joins the optic nerve from the other

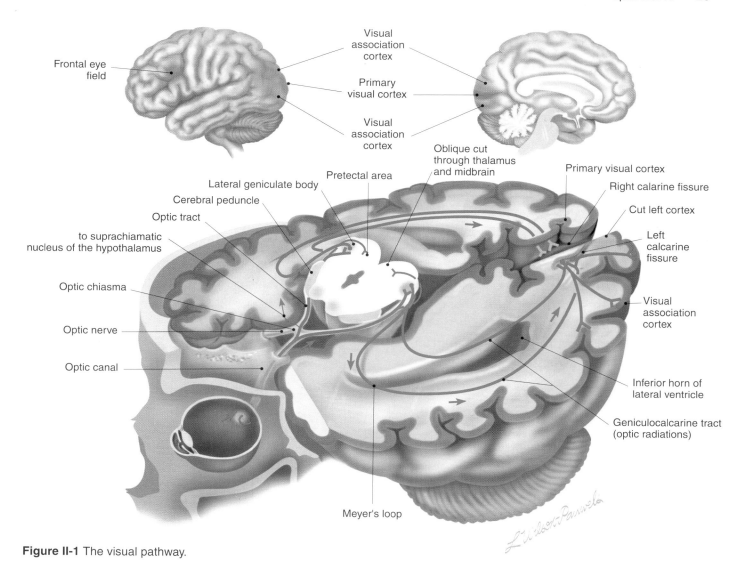

Frontal eye field

Visual association cortex

Primary visual cortex

Visual association cortex

Oblique cut through thalamus and midbrain

Pretectal area

Lateral geniculate body

Cerebral peduncle

Optic tract

to suprachiamatic nucleus of the hypothalamus

Optic chiasma

Optic nerve

Optic canal

Primary visual cortex

Right calarine fissure

Cut left cortex

Left calcarine fissure

Visual association cortex

Inferior horn of lateral ventricle

Geniculocalcarine tract (optic radiations)

Meyer's loop

Figure II-1 The visual pathway.

Note that the optic nerve, like the olfactory nerve, is composed of secondary sensory axons rather than primary sensory axons and so forms a central nervous system tract rather than a nerve. Nevertheless, the part of the tract that runs from the eye to the chiasma is known as the optic "nerve."

eye to form the optic chiasma (literally the "optic cross"). A small number of axons from each eye leave the chiasma and course superiorly to the suprachiasmatic nucleus of the hypothalamus where they act to influence the circadian rhythm. At the chiasma, approximately one-half of the axons cross the midline to join the uncrossed axons from the other eye, forming the optic tracts. The optic tracts continue posteriorly around the cerebral peduncles. A small number of the axons in each tract terminate in the pretectal area of the midbrain where they form the afferent limb of the pupillary light reflex. The remaining axons terminate in the lateral geniculate body (nucleus) of the thalamus.

Axons of lateral geniculate neurons form the geniculocalcarine tract (optic radiations). They enter the cerebral hemisphere through the sublenticular part of the internal capsule, fan out above and lateral to the inferior horn of the lateral ventricle, and course posteriorly to terminate in the primary visual cortex surrounding the calcarine fissure. A proportion of these axons form Meyer's loop by coursing anteriorly toward the pole of the temporal lobe before turning posteriorly.

From the primary visual cortex, integrated visual signals are sent to the adjacent visual association areas for interpretation and to the frontal eye fields (see Figure II–1) where they direct changes in visual fixation.

Table II–1 Nerve Fiber Modality and Function of the Optic Nerve

Nerve Fiber Modality	Function
Special sensory (afferent)	To convey visual information from the retina

ANATOMY OF THE RETINA

The retina is a specialized sensory structure that lines the posterior half of each eye. The central point of the retina is called the macula (spot), in the center of which lies the fovea (pit) (Figures II–2 and II–3). The area of the retina medial to the fovea is called the nasal hemiretina (close to the nose) and that lateral to the fovea is the temporal hemiretina (close to the temporal bone). An imaginary horizontal line through the fovea further divides the retina into upper and lower halves. The optic disk lies in the nasal hemiretina just above the horizontal meridian. Optic nerve axons leave the eye, and blood vessels enter the eye at the optic disk. There are no photoreceptors in the optic disk; therefore, it forms a blind spot in the visual field.

The vertebrate retina is inverted (ie, the photoreceptors are at the back of the retina not at the front where light rays first strike). Photons (light energy) transverse all the cellular layers of the retina, including the blood vessels that supply it, before they encounter the photoreceptors (see Figure II–3). The fovea is the area of the

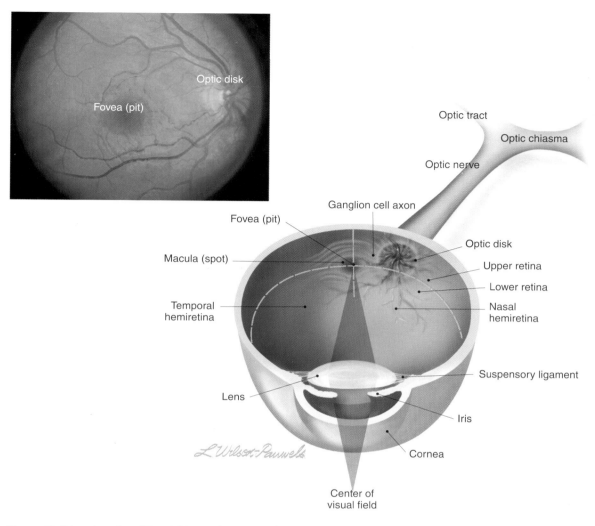

Figure II–2 Landmarks of the right eye demonstrating ganglion cell axons diverting around the macula. (Fundus photograph courtesy of Dr. R. Buncic.)

retina that provides high-resolution central vision. It has several anatomic features that facilitate the passage of photons to the photoreceptors.

1. Most ganglion cell axons take the most direct path toward the optic disk; however, those whose direct route would take them across the front of the fovea, divert around it so as not to interfere with central vision (see Figure II–2).

2. The fovea is avascular (ie, there are no capillaries in front of the photoreceptors to deflect the light rays). The photoreceptors in the fovea are supplied with oxygen and nutrients by a dense bed of capillaries behind the pigmented epithelium (see Figure II–3).

3. The layers of the retina thin out at the fovea such that there are only a single layer of photoreceptors and a few cells of Müller (retinal glial cells) (see Figure II–3).

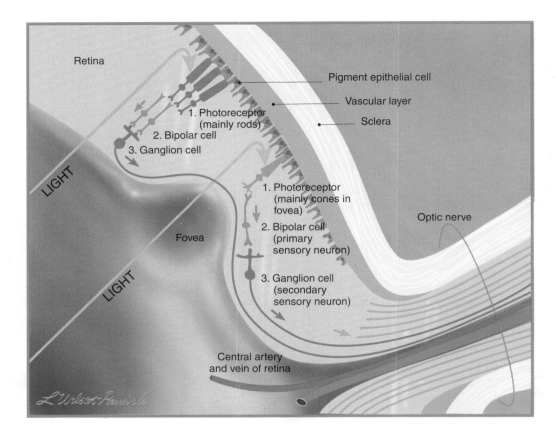

Figure II–3 Retinal layers (enlarged for clarity).

Light entering the eye travels through the pupil and passes to the back of the retina to reach the photoreceptor layer (rods and cones) where light energy is transduced into electrical signals.* The information received by the photoreceptors is passed forward in the retina to the bipolar cells, which pass the signal further forward to ganglion cells in the anterior layers of the retina. Ganglion cell axons converge toward the optic disk, turn posteriorly, pass through the lamina cribriformis of the sclera, and leave the eye as the optic nerve (see Figure II–3). Considerable processing of the retinal signal takes place within the middle layers of the retina.

Photoreceptors

Photoreceptors are specialized neurons with all the usual cellular components and, in addition, a light-sensitive outer segment composed of stacked layers of membrane (disks) that contain visual pigments. The disks are continuously produced in the

---

*Details of signal processing in the retina are beyond the scope of this text; however, the interested reader can find excellent descriptions in Wurtz RH, Kandel ER. Central visual pathways. In: Kandel ER, Schwartz JH, Jessell TM, editors. Principles of neural science. 4th ed. New York: McGraw Hill; 2000. p. 523–47; and Reid RC. Vision. In: Zigmond MJ, Bloom FE, Landis SC, et al, editors. Fundamental neuroscience. San Diego: Academic Press; 1999. p. 821–51.

inner segment. Approximately 10 percent of the disks at the distal end are shed daily and phagocytosed by the pigment epithelial cells; therefore, the outer segment is completely replaced about every 10 days. There are two types of photoreceptors: rods and cones (Figure II–4).

Rods function in dim light. They have about 700 disks containing a high concentration of rhodopsin, which makes them highly sensitive to light. They are capable of detecting a single photon; however, they saturate in bright light and are not used in daytime vision. There are approximately 130 million rods in each human retina. They constitute most of the photoreceptors in the peripheral retina and are almost absent in the fovea. There is a high degree of convergence of rods to ganglion cells and only one kind of rod pigment; therefore, the rod system produces low resolution achromatic vision.

Cones function in bright light. The number of disks in their outer segments varies from a few hundred in the peripheral retina to over 1,000 in the fovea; however, they have less photopigment than the rods and are therefore less sensitive to light. Cone cells are of three types according to their maximal spectral sensitivities: red, green, and blue. They are, therefore, responsible for color vision. Cones are not active in dim light, which is why colors seem to disappear at dusk. There are approximately 7 million cones (far fewer than the number of rods). They are present in very low numbers in the peripheral retina, but are found in high densities in the central part of the retina and are almost the only photoreceptors in the central fovea.

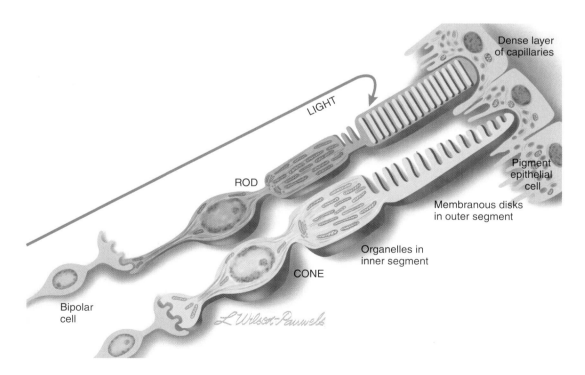

Figure II–4 Photoreceptor cells of the retina.

Ganglion Cells

Ganglion cells receive signals from the photoreceptors via bipolar cells and send signals to the lateral geniculate bodies. There are approximately 137 photoreceptors for each ganglion cell; therefore, there is considerable convergence of signals. The number of photoreceptors that converge on a single ganglion cell varies from several thousand in the periphery of the retina to one in the central fovea (Figure II–5). This one-to-one projection in the fovea provides for the high resolution in central vision (see Figure II–5A). Approximately half the ganglion cell axons in the optic nerve represent the fovea and the region just around it. Furthermore, half the primary visual cortex surrounding the calcarine fissure represents the fovea and the area just around it (Figure II–6).

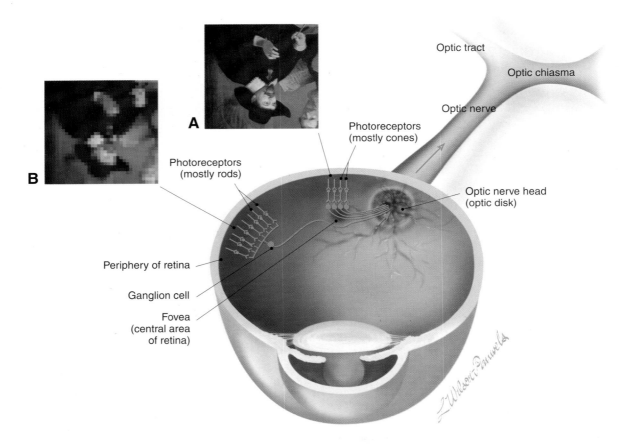

Figure II–5 Convergence of photoreceptors on ganglion cells: several thousand to one at the periphery of the retina and one to one at the fovea. The retinal layer is exaggerated for clarity. *A,* Demonstrates high resolution and color in the fovea. *B,* Demonstrates low resolution and poor color in the peripheral retina. The image on the retina is upside down and laterally reversed. (Detail from Rembrant's *The Anatomy Lesson of Dr. Tulp.*)

There are two major classes of ganglion cells: M cells (magni–large) and P cells (parvi–small). The M cells respond optimally to large objects and are able to follow rapid changes in the stimulus. They are, therefore, specialized for detecting motion. The P cells are more numerous, respond selectively to specific wavelengths, and are involved in the perception of form and color. An easy way to remember the difference is M stands for magni and movement and P stands for parvi and particulars. These differences in function are due to both the physiologic differences in the ganglion cells themselves and to their connections with other cells in the retina.

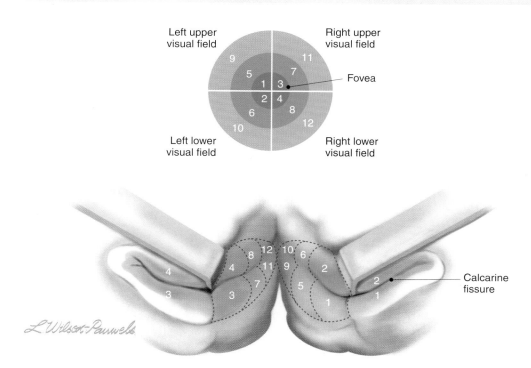

Figure II–6 The primary visual cortices surrounding the calcarine fissures receive signals from the four quadrants of the visual fields. The upper visual fields are mapped below the calcarine fissures and the lower visual fields are mapped above the calcarine fissures. The posterior half of the primary visual cortex receives signals from the fovea and surrounding area.

TRANSMISSION OF INFORMATION FROM VARIOUS PARTS OF THE VISUAL FIELD

The visual field is defined as everything we see without moving our head. The visual field has both binocular (seen with two eyes) and monocular (seen with one eye) zones. Light from the binocular zone strikes the retina in both eyes. Light from the monocular zone strikes the retina in the ipsilateral eye only; its access to the contralateral eye is limited by the nose and by the size of the contralateral pupil. Normally, both eyes focus on the same object and view the same visual field but from slightly different angles because of the separation of the eyes. It is this separation that provides depth perception.

Rays of light from the visual fields converge, pass through the relatively small pupil, and are refracted by the lens before they reach the retinae. As a result, the visual fields are projected onto the retinae both upside down and laterally reversed (Figure II–7). Ganglion cell axons carrying visual information from the four retinal quadrants converge toward the optic disk in an orderly fashion and maintain

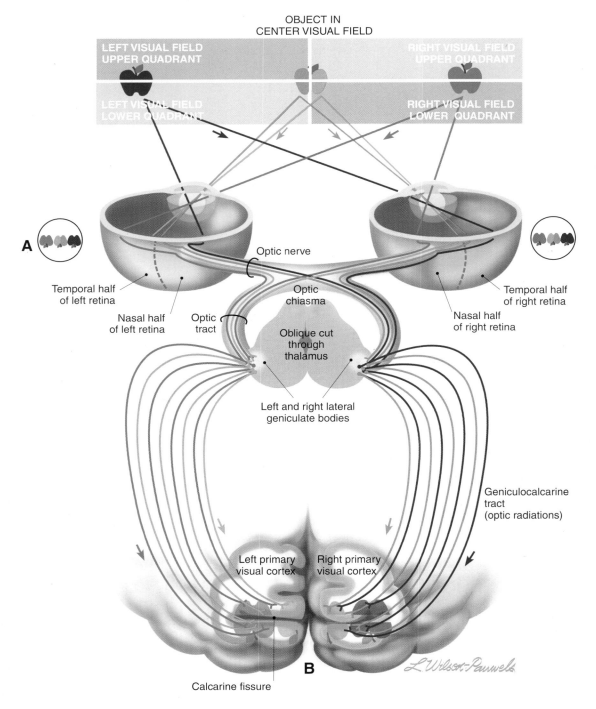

Figure II–7 *A,* Projection of the visual field onto the retinae upside down and laterally reversed. *B,* Transmission of signals from the left and right visual fields from **both** eyes to the contralateral visual cortices.

approximately the same relationship to each other within the optic nerve (see Figure II–5). Within the chiasma, axons from the nasal halves of both retinae cross the midline. This arrangement of axons results in the information from the right half of the visual field from both eyes being carried in the left optic tract and the left half of the visual field from both eyes being carried in the right optic tract.

From the lateral geniculate bodies (nuclei), information from the upper halves of the retinae (lower visual field) is carried to the cortices that form the upper wall of the calcarine fissure. Information from the lower halves of the retinae (upper visual field) terminates in the cortices that form the lower walls of the calcarine fissure (Figure II–8).

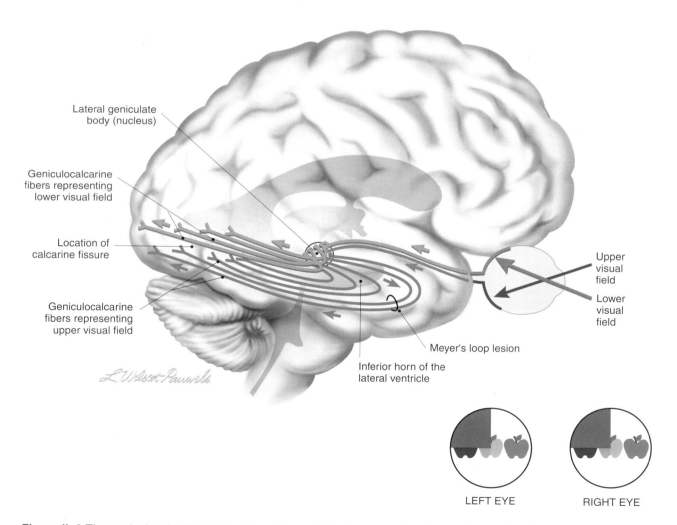

Figure II–8 The geniculocalcarine tracts viewed through the transparent surface of the brain. Information from the upper retina (lower visual field) projects to the cortex surrounding the upper wall of the calcarine fissure and information from the lower retina (upper visual field) projects to the cortex surrounding the lower wall of the fissure. *Circle insets,* A lesion of right Meyer's loop axons results in a loss of vision in the upper contralateral (left) visual quadrants—homonymous quadrantanopia (for other visual pathway lesions see page 42).

The eyes are constantly scanning the visual field. The retina sends signals to the primary visual cortex (see Figure II–6), which constructs a representation of the visual field (Figure II–9A). Signals from the primary visual cortex are sent continuously to the visual association cortex for further processing. These signals are used to construct a perceived visual field that is right side up and oriented correctly from left to right. The resolution is perceived to be constant across the field (Figure II–9B).

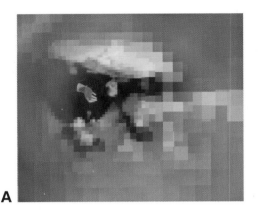
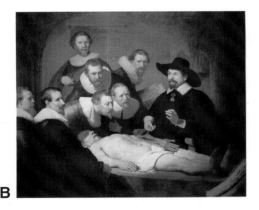

Figure II–9 *A,* How the retina sees the visual field; upside down and laterally reversed with decreasing resolution and decreasing color discrimination from the fovea outward. Focus is on the doctor's left hand. *B,* How higher cortical areas reconstruct the visual field. (Detail from Rembrant's *The Anatomy Lesson of Dr. Tulp.*)

CASE HISTORY GUIDING QUESTIONS

1. Why is Meredith's vision blurred?

2. What is the pupillary light reflex?

3. Why was there little constriction of Meredith's pupils when a bright light was shone in her right eye?

4. What other lesions of the visual pathway result in visual loss?

1. Why is Meredith's vision blurred?

The resolution in the central retina only (fovea) is high enough to allow for reading and recognition of faces (Figures II–9A and II–10A). The inflammation in Meredith's right optic nerve (optic neuritis) interferes with transmission of signals from the retina to the brain stem. Because a high proportion of the optic nerve axons originate in the fovea, Meredith's central vision is considerably compromised, and vision in her right eye is therefore blurry (Figure II–10B).

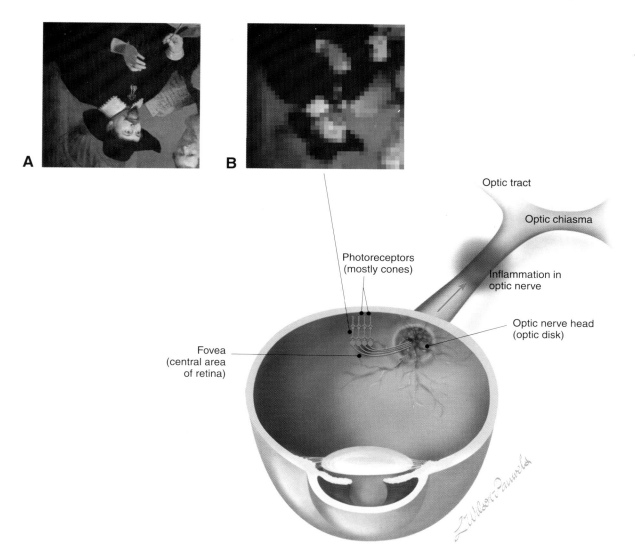

Figure II–10 *A,* Normally Meredith's central vision has high acuity and color infomation. *B,* Inflammation in her right optic nerve interferes with the transmission of signals from the retina to the brain. Since half the axons in the optic nerve carry signals from the fovea, the major change Meredith perceives is a loss of acuity and color in her central vision. (Detail from Rembrant's *The Anatomy Lesson of Dr. Tulp.*)

Optic neuritis is inflammation of the optic nerve. It occurs more commonly in women than in men and in younger patients, 20 to 50 years old. Visual loss is typically monocular and progresses over hours to days. This is frequently associated with ocular pain on eye movement, central visual loss, decreased visual acuity, altered color vision, and an afferent pupillary defect.

2. What is the pupillary light reflex?

Very bright light damages the retina. The pupillary light reflex evolved to control the amount of light entering the eye. In dim light the pupil is dilated to allow maximal entry of light, however, as the light gets brighter the pupil gets smaller. The pupillary light reflex involves two cranial nerves: the optic nerve (cranial nerve II) forms the afferent limb by carrying the sensory signal to the central nervous system, and the oculomotor nerve (cranial nerve III) forms the efferent limb by carrying motor signals to the pupillary constrictor muscle.

Light entering the eyes causes signals to be sent along the optic nerves to the Edinger-Westphal nuclei in the pretectal region of the midbrain. Visceral motor signals arising in these nuclei are sent along preganglionic parasympathetic axons in the oculomotor nerves to the ciliary ganglia. Postganglionic axons leave the ciliary ganglia via six to ten short ciliary nerves to enter the eyes at their posterior aspects near the exit of the optic nerves. Within the eyeball, the nerves run forward between the choroid and sclera to terminate in the constrictor pupillae muscles of the iris (Figure II–11).

In the normal reflex, light shone in either eye causes constriction of the pupil in the same eye (the direct light reflex) and also in the other eye (the consensual light reflex).

> The pupillary light reflex is used to assess the function of the brain stem in a comatose patient and is one of the brain stem reflexes tested in the determination of brain death.

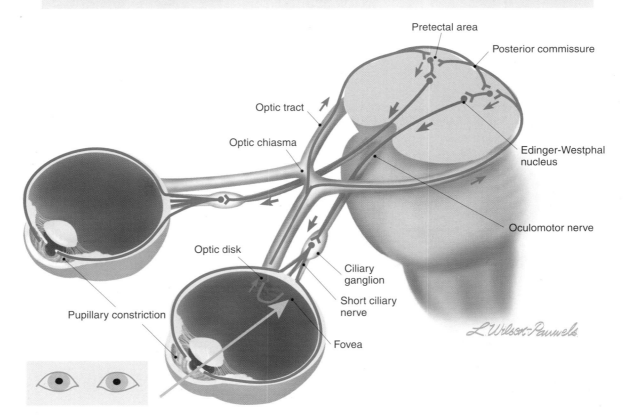

Figure II–11 Pupillary light reflex. Light shone in Meredith's left eye causes direct (left) and consensual (right) pupillary constriction.

3. Why was there little constriction of Meredith's pupils when a bright light was shone in her right eye?

When a light was shone into Meredith's right eye, transmission of the signal to her midbrain was reduced or blocked because of inflammation of the optic nerve. The defect in the afferent limb of the reflex pathway resulted in poor direct and consensual pupillary responses relative to the response produced by light shone in the intact eye. This is referred to as a relative afferent pupillary defect (Figure II–12). Compare Meredith's afferent pupillary defect with Werner's efferent pupillary defect in Chapter III, Figure III–11.

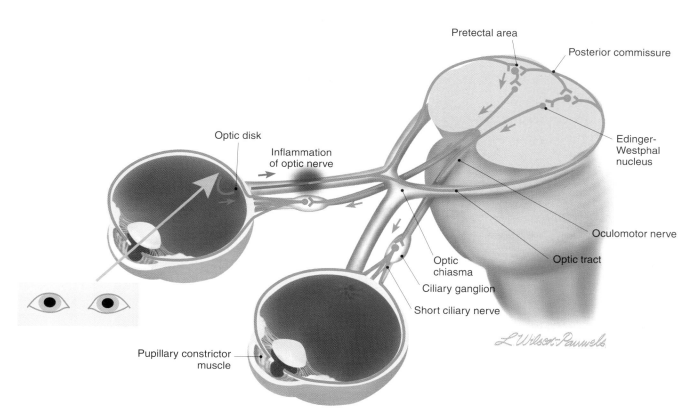

Figure II–12 Relative afferent pupillary defect. Light shone in Meredith's right eye results in the absence of direct (right) and consensual (left) pupillary constriction.

4. What other lesions of the visual pathway result in visual loss?

Lesions in different sites in the optic pathway produce different patterns of visual loss. Typical sites for damage and the visual loss that each produces are shown in Figures II–13 to II–15.

Clinically it is useful to group visual pathway lesions into three categories:

1. *Anterior to the Chiasma*
   Damage to the light-transmitting parts of the eye, the retina, or the optic nerve results in visual loss in the affected eye only (monocular visual loss) (eg, see Figure II–13).

2. *At the Chiasma*
   Damage to the optic chiasma usually results in loss of vision from both eyes, depending on which axons are affected (bitemporal hemianopia) (eg, see Figure II–14).

3. *Posterior to the Chiasma*
   Damage to the optic tracts, lateral geniculate body, optic radiations, or visual cortices results in visual loss from both eyes within the contralateral visual field (homonymous hemianopia) (eg, see Figures II–8B and II–15). Because input from the fovea occupies such a large proportion of the axons in the optic radiations, most lesions posterior to the lateral geniculate bodies generally do not eliminate all central vision unless the lesion is a massive one. This phenomenon is called macular sparing (remember that the macula is the area of the central retina that includes the fovea).

Lesions that involve only a subgroup of axons in the visual pathway produce scotomas (ie, partial loss of the visual field). Scotomas are also called blind spots. Meredith has a scotoma in her right eye.

Remember that the visual fields are projected onto the retinae upside down and laterally reversed. Therefore, damage to the right sides of the retinae or to the neurons that receive signals from them will result in perceived defects in the left visual field and vice versa. Similarly, damage to the upper halves of the retinae or to the neurons that receive signals from them will result in defects in the lower visual field and vice versa.

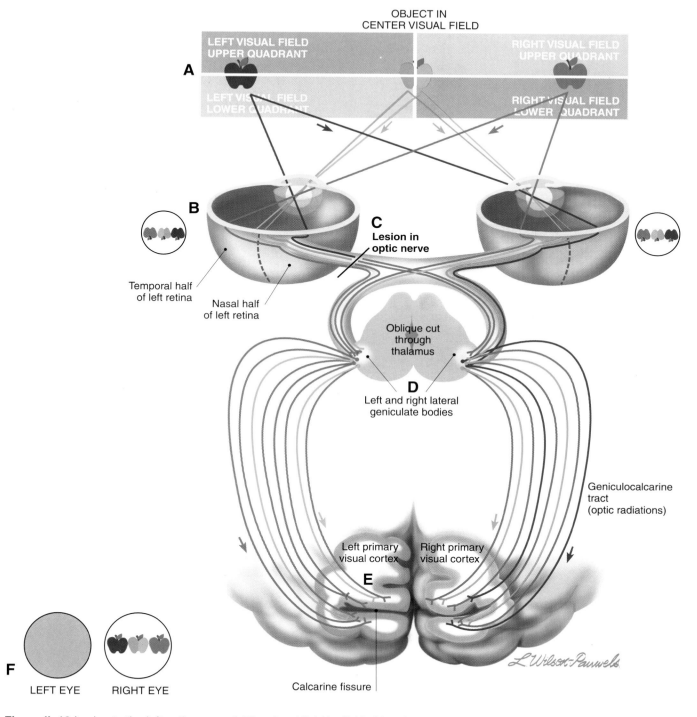

Figure II–13 Lesion to the left optic nerve. *A,* The visual field is divided into four quadrants that are *B,* projected upside down and laterally reversed onto the retinae. *C,* An optic nerve lesion interrupts signals from the left temporal and nasal hemiretina to the *D,* lateral geniculate bodies resulting in *E,* the primary visual cortices only receiving input from the right eye. *F,* As a result, the patient is blind in his left eye (monocular visual loss).

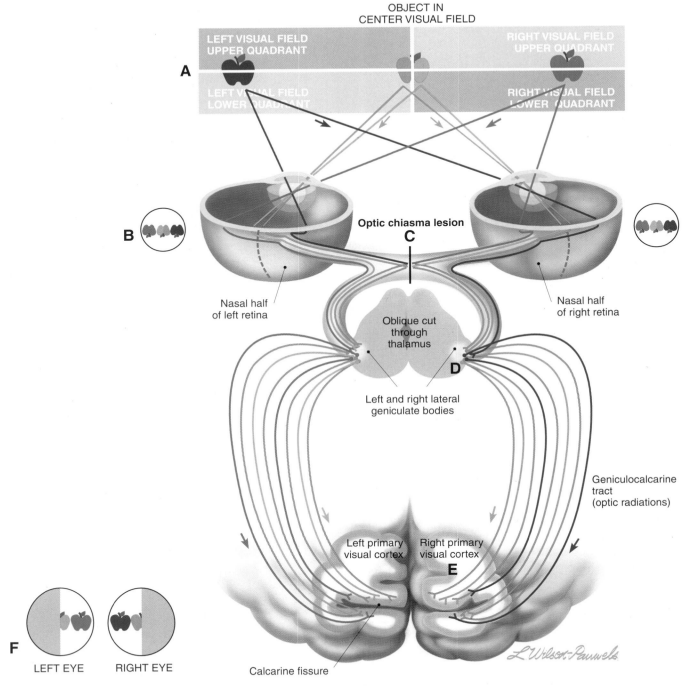

OBJECT IN
CENTER VISUAL FIELD

LEFT VISUAL FIELD
UPPER QUADRANT

RIGHT VISUAL FIELD
UPPER QUADRANT

A

LEFT VISUAL FIELD
LOWER QUADRANT

RIGHT VISUAL FIELD
LOWER QUADRANT

Optic chiasma lesion
C

B

Nasal half
of left retina

Nasal half
of right retina

Oblique cut
through
thalamus

D

Left and right lateral
geniculate bodies

Geniculocalcarine
tract
(optic radiations)

Left primary
visual cortex

Right primary
visual cortex

E

F

LEFT EYE   RIGHT EYE

Calcarine fissure

L. Wilson-Pauwels

Figure II–14 Lesion of the optic chiasma. *A,* The visual field is divided into four quadrants that are *B,* projected upside down and laterally reversed onto the retinae. *C,* A lesion of the midline of the optic chiasma interrupts the transmission of signals from the left and right nasal hemiretinae to the *D,* left and right lateral geniculate bodies. These retinal halves view the temporal visual fields; therefore, no visual stimuli from the temporal fields reach the *E,* primary visual cortices. *F,* As a result, the patient loses peripheral vision (bitemporal hemianopia).

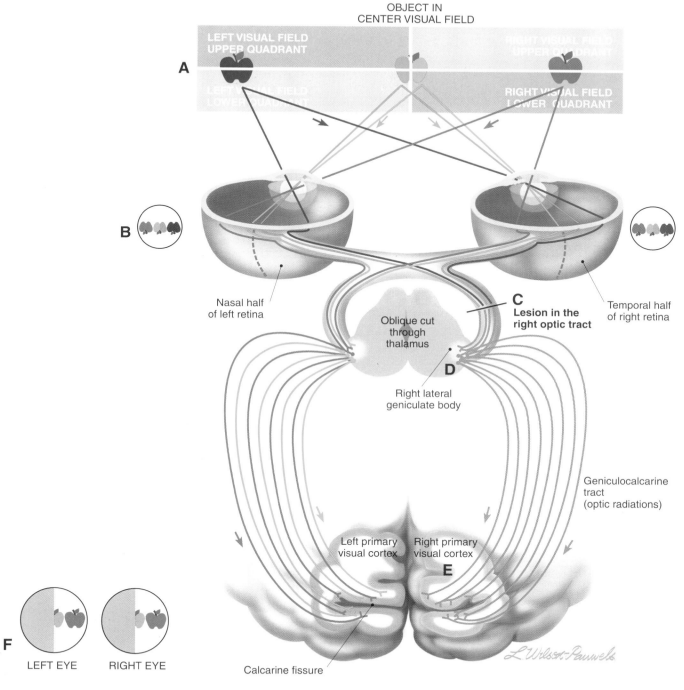

Figure II–15 Lesion to the right optic tract. *A,* The visual field is divided into four quadrants that are *B,* projected upside down and laterally reversed onto the retinae. *C,* A right optic tract lesion interrupts signals from the left nasal hemiretina and the right temporal hemiretina to the *D,* right lateral geniculate body. *E,* Both of these retinal halves view the left visual field; therefore, no visual stimuli from the left visual field reach the right primary visual cortex. *F,* This visual defect is called homonymous (same side) hemianopia and results in blindness in the left half of the visual field in both eyes.

CLINICAL TESTING

Examination of the optic nerve involves four procedures:

1. Visualization of the fundus

2. Measurement of visual acuity

3. Testing of visual fields

4. Testing of the pupillary light reflex

(See also Cranial Nerves Examination on CD-ROM.)

Visualization of the Fundus

Visualization of the fundus (Figure II–16) involves the use of an ophthalmoscope. The examination is performed in a dimly lit room so that the patient's pupils are maximally dilated. Ask the patient to focus on an object in the distance. This helps to keep the eyes still and allows for better visualization of the fundus. The first thing to look at is the disk (optic nerve head). The margins of the disk should be sharp. Blurring of the disk margins is seen with raised intracranial pressure, and disk pallor is an indication of optic atrophy. You should also note the optic cup. The optic cup is a depression in the center of the disk from which vessels emerge. Take a close look at the vessels, venous pulsations can be seen in 85 to 90 percent of patients. They disappear if the intracranial pressure is raised. Lastly, look at the retina and macula for further evidence of disease. Ophthalmoscopy takes a lot of practice and we recommend that you practice on your classmates to become familiar with the appearance of a normal fundus.

Measurement of Visual Acuity

Visual acuity is best assessed using Snellen's chart (Figure II–17) at 6 feet; however, a hand-held visual acuity card can be used at the bedside. The patient may wear his

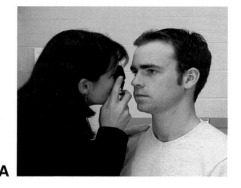
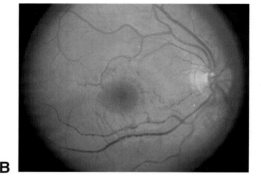

Figure II–16 Examination of the fundus. *A,* The physician is examining the patient's right fundus using an ophthalmoscope. *B,* Normal fundus of the right eye. (Fundus photograph courtesy of Dr. R. Buncic.)

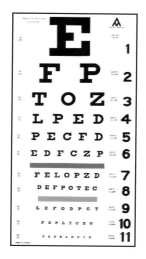 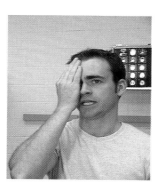

Figure II–17 Visual acuity is tested using Snellen's chart.

or her glasses, and each eye is tested separately. Visual acuity is a test of macular function. The macula gives rise to the majority of the optic nerve fibers; therefore, inflammation or a lesion of the optic nerve can result in significant loss of visual acuity.

Testing of Visual Fields

Visual field testing (Figure II–18) at the bed side involves comparison of the examiner's visual fields with those of the patient. Sit directly across from the patient. Instruct the patient to focus on your nose and then ask the patient to close his left eye. You, in turn, close your right eye and, with your arm fully extended, bring your index finger from beyond the periphery of vision toward the center of the visual field (see Figure II–18B). The patient is asked to indicate when the finger is first seen. Both you and the patient should see the finger at the same time. Your finger should be brought in obliquely in all four quadrants. The procedure is repeated for the other

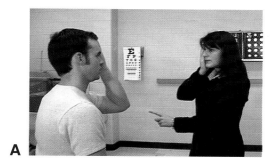 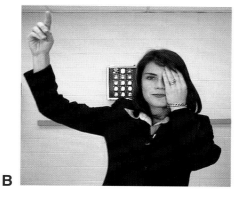

Figure II–18 Testing of the visual field. *A,* Testing the lower left quadrant of the patient's right eye (patient's left eye and physician's right eye are covered). *B,* Patient's view of the physician testing the upper left quadrant of the patient's left eye (patient's right eye and physician's left eye are covered).

eye. A field defect is likely present if the patient fails to see your finger once it is in your own visual field.

A full understanding of the anatomy of the visual pathway is necessary to interpret the results of visual field testing (see Figures II–1 and II–8).

Testing of the Pupillary Light Reflex

The pupillary light reflex relies on the integrity of both cranial nerve II (the afferent pathway) and the parasympathetic nerve fibers that travel with cranial nerve III (the efferent pathway). A beam of light is shone directly on one pupil. If both the afferent and efferent pathways are intact, the ipsilateral pupil constricts; this is the direct response. The contralateral pupil should also constrict. This is the indirect (consensual) response (see Figure II–11).

ADDITIONAL RESOURCES

Ebers GC. Optic neuritis and multiple sclerosis. Arch Neurol 1985;42:702–4.

Kurtzke JF. Optic neuritis and multiple sclerosis. Arch Neurol 1985;42:704–10.

Optic Neuritis Study Group. The clinical profile of optic neuritis. Arch Ophthalmol 1991;109:1673–8.

Pryse-Phillips W. Companion to clinical neurology. 1st ed. Toronto: Little, Brown and Co.; 1995. p. 639.

Reid RC. Vision. In: Zigmond MJ, Bloom FE, Landis SC, et al, editors. Fundamental neuroscience. San Diego: Academic Press; 1999. p. 821–51.

Warren LA. Basic anatomy of the human eye for artists. J Biocommun 1988;15(1):22–30.

Wurtz RH, Kandel ER. Central visual pathways. In: Kandel ER, Schwartz JH, Jessell TM, editors. Principles of neural science. 4th ed. New York: McGraw-Hill; 2000. p. 523–47.

III Oculomotor Nerve

innervates four of the six extrinsic ocular muscles and the intrinsic ocular muscles

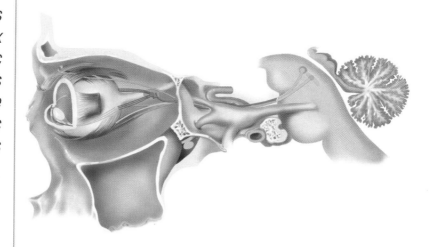

III Oculomotor Nerve

CASE HISTORY

Werner is a 54-year-old gentleman whose favorite pastime is working in his garden. One afternoon, while lifting a heavy potted plant, he experienced a sudden headache. This headache was the worst he had ever experienced and he started to vomit. Concerned about the headache's sudden nature and intensity, he went to the emergency department.

In the emergency department, Werner was drowsy and had a stiff neck, although he was rousable and able to answer questions and follow commands. When a bright light was shone into his left eye, his left pupil constricted briskly, but the right pupil remained dilated. When the light was shone directly into his right eye, his right pupil remained dilated and his left pupil constricted. Werner also had a droopy right eyelid, and when he was asked to look straight ahead, his right eye deviated slightly down and to the right. Werner complained of double vision and recalled that he had experienced some sensitivity to light in his right eye during the two weeks preceding this event. Close examination of Werner's eye movements revealed that he could move his left eye in all directions, but had difficulty with movements of his right eye. With his right eye, Werner was able to look to the right (abduct) but he could not look to the left (adduct). He was unable to look directly up or down. Werner's other cranial nerves were tested and found to be functioning normally.

The emergency physician was concerned that Werner might have experienced a subarachnoid hemorrhage. A computed tomography (CT) scan of his head was done, and this demonstrated blood in the subarachnoid space. A cerebral angiogram was done, which demonstrated a dilated aneurysm of the right posterior communicating artery. Werner subsequently underwent neurosurgery to have the aneurysm clipped.

ANATOMY OF THE OCULOMOTOR NERVE

As its name implies, the oculomotor nerve plays a major role in eye movement (Table III–1). Its somatic motor component innervates four of the six extraocular (extrinsic) muscles and its visceral motor component innervates the intrinsic ocular muscles (constrictor pupillae and the ciliary muscle). The nerve also innervates the levator palpebrae superioris muscle, which elevates the upper eyelid.

The oculomotor nerve emerges from the interpeduncular fossa on the ventral aspect of the midbrain (Figure III–1). After passing between the posterior cerebral and superior cerebellar arteries, the nerve courses anteriorly. It pierces the dura and enters the cavernous sinus (Figure III–2) where it runs along the lateral wall of the sinus just superior to the trochlear nerve (cranial nerve IV) and then continues forward through the superior orbital fissure. As the oculomotor nerve enters the orbit through the tendinous ring, it splits into superior and inferior divisions.

Table III–1 Nerve Fiber Modality and Function of the Oculomotor Nerve

Nerve Fiber Modality	Nucleus	Function
Somatic motor (efferent)	Oculomotor	Innervation of the levator palpebrae superioris, superior, medial, and inferior recti, and inferior oblique muscles of the eye
Visceral motor (parasympathetic efferent)	Edinger-Westphal	Parasympathetic supply to constrictor pupillae and ciliary muscles

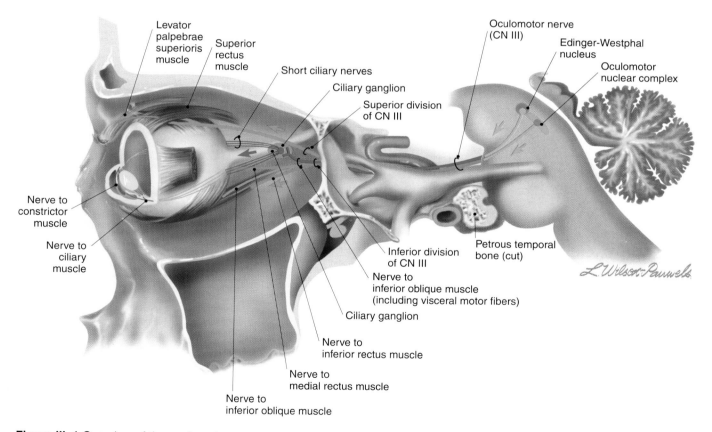

Figure III–1 Overview of the oculomotor nerve.

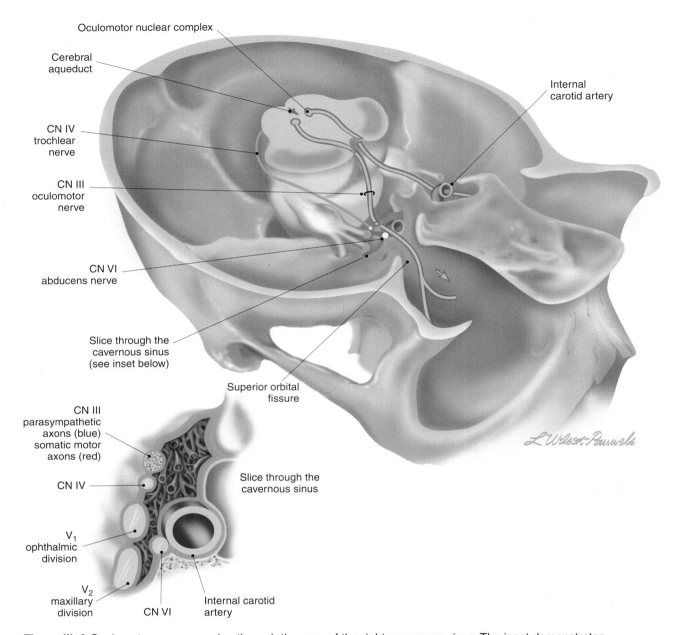

Figure III–2 Oculomotor nerve coursing through the area of the right cavernous sinus. The inset demonstrates the anatomic relationships of the structures coursing through the cavernous sinus. Note in cranial nerve III the parasympathetic axons are located on the surface of the nerve.

The superior division innervates the superior rectus and the levator palpebrae superioris muscles. The inferior division innnervates the medial rectus, inferior rectus, and inferior oblique muscles. The visceral motor axons run with the nerve to the inferior oblique muscle for a short distance, then leave it to terminate in the ciliary ganglion. Postganglionic axons leave the ciliary ganglion as eight to ten short ciliary nerves to enter the eye at the posterior aspect near the exit of the optic nerve (see Figure III–1).

The oculomotor nucleus is situated in the midbrain at the level of the superior colliculus. Like the other somatic motor nuclei, the oculomotor nucleus is near the midline. It is located just ventral to the cerebral aqueduct and is bounded laterally and inferiorly by the medial longitudinal fasciculus. It is generally accepted that sub-nuclei within the oculomotor complex supply individual muscles (Figure III–3).

The lateral part of the oculomotor complex is formed by the lateral subnuclei, which, from dorsal to ventral and ipsilaterally, supply the inferior rectus, inferior oblique, and medial rectus muscles. The medial subnucleus supplies the contralateral superior rectus muscle, and the central subnucleus (a midline mass of cells at the caudal end of the complex) supplies the levators palpebrae superioris, bilaterally.

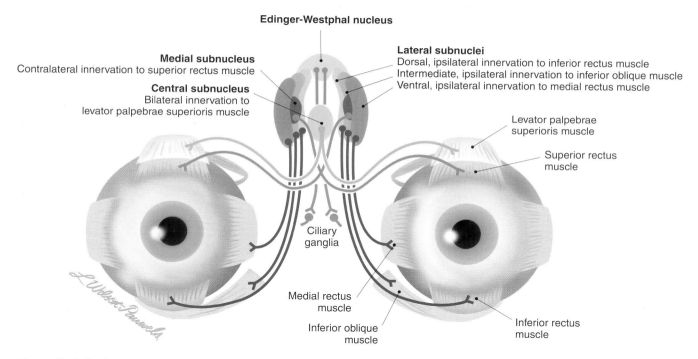

Edinger-Westphal nucleus

Medial subnucleus
Contralateral innervation to superior rectus muscle

Central subnucleus
Bilateral innervation to
levator palpebrae superioris muscle

Lateral subnuclei
Dorsal, ipsilateral innervation to inferior rectus muscle
Intermediate, ipsilateral innervation to inferior oblique muscle
Ventral, ipsilateral innervation to medial rectus muscle

Levator palpebrae
superioris muscle

Superior rectus
muscle

Ciliary
ganglia

Medial rectus
muscle

Inferior oblique
muscle

Inferior rectus
muscle

Figure III–3 Oculomotor nuclear complex and schematic innervation of extraocular muscles (the functions of the Edinger-Westphal nucleus are discussed with the visceral motor component of cranial nerve III).

SOMATIC MOTOR (EFFERENT) COMPONENT

Somatic motor neuron axons leave the oculomotor nuclear complex and course ventrally in the tegmentum of the midbrain through the medial portion of the red nucleus and the medial aspect of the cerebral peduncle to emerge in the interpeduncular fossa at the junction between the midbrain and the pons (see Figure III–2).

As the somatic motor axons enter the orbital cavity through the superior orbital fissure, they branch into superior and inferior divisions (Figure III–4). The superior division ascends lateral to the optic nerve to supply the superior rectus and levator palpebrae superioris muscles. The inferior division divides into three branches that supply the inferior rectus, inferior oblique, and medial rectus muscles. The muscles are innervated on their ocular surfaces, except for the inferior oblique, whose branch enters the posterior border of the muscle (Figure III–5).

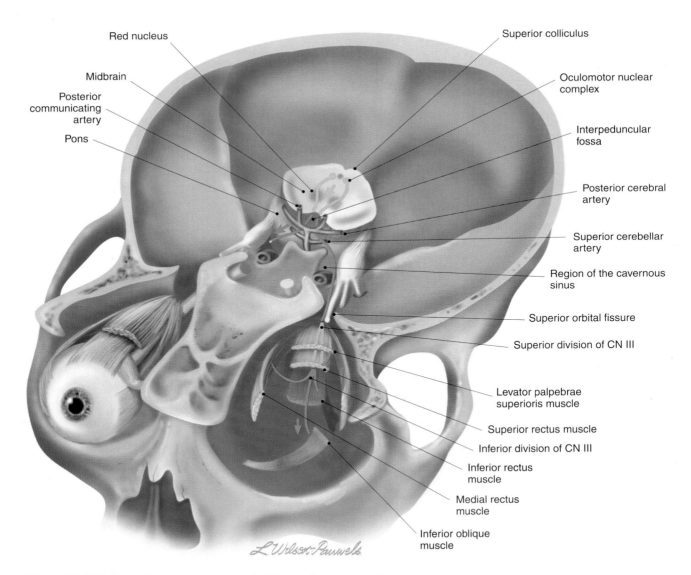

Figure III–4 The somatic motor component of the oculomotor nerve.

Table III–2 summarizes the actions of the muscles supplied by cranial nerve III that move the eye.

Table III–2 Eye Movements Mediated by Cranial Nerve III

Nerve	Muscle(s)	Primary action(s)	Secondary action(s)
CN III	Medial rectus	Adduction	None
	Inferior rectus	Downward gaze	Extorsion
	Superior rectus	Upward gaze	Intorsion
	Inferior oblique	Upward gaze	Abduction and extorsion

In addition, cranial nerve III innervates the levator palpebrae superioris muscle, which raises the eyelid during upward gaze (see Figure III–5).

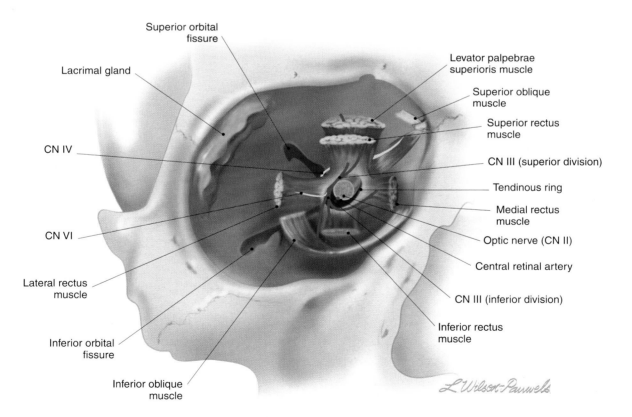

Figure III–5 Apex of the right orbit, illustrating the tendinous ring and the somatic motor component of cranial nerve III.

The primary action of the medial rectus muscle is to adduct the eye toward the nose, the inferior rectus muscle turns the eye downward and extorts it, and the superior rectus muscle rolls the eye upward and intorts it. The inferior oblique muscle rolls the eye upward and abducts and extorts it. The combinations of these muscles, plus the superior oblique (cranial nerve IV) and lateral rectus (cranial nerve VI) muscles, enable eye movement around the three axes of the eye (Figure III–6).

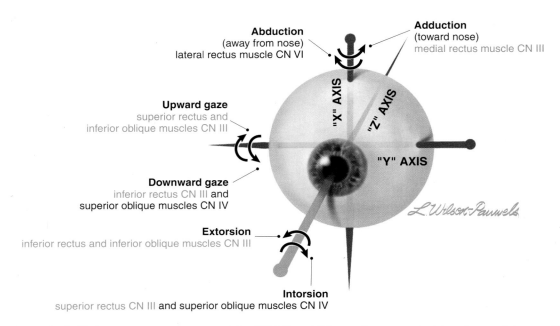

Figure III–6   Right eye movements around the "X," "Y," and "Z" axes (movements driven by cranial nerve III are highlighted in pink).

VISCERAL MOTOR (PARASYMPATHETIC EFFERENT) COMPONENT

The Edinger-Westphal (visceral motor) nucleus is located in the midbrain, dorsal to the anterior portion of the oculomotor complex (see Figures III–1 and III–3). Preganglionic visceral motor axons leave the nucleus and course ventrally through the midbrain with the somatic motor axons. The parasympathetic and somatic axons together constitute cranial nerve III. The parasympathetic axons are located on the surface of the nerve. Therefore, when the nerve is compressed, the parasympathetic axons are the first axons to lose their function (see Figure III–2). The parasympathetic axons branch from the nerve to the inferior oblique muscle and terminate in the ciliary ganglion near the apex of the cone of extraocular muscles (see Figure III–1).

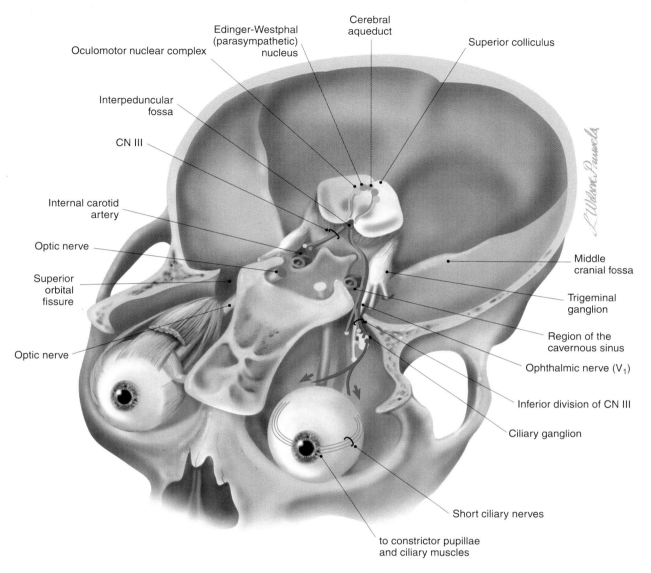

Figure III–7 The visceral motor component of the oculomotor nerve travels with the somatic motor axons that form the inferior division of cranial nerve III (roof of skull and orbit removed).

Postganglionic axons leave the ciliary ganglion as six to ten short ciliary nerves to enter the eye at its posterior aspect near the origin of the optic nerve. Within the eyeball, the nerves run forward, between the choroid and the sclera, to terminate in the ciliary body and the constrictor pupillae muscle (Figure III–7).

The visceral motor fibers control the tone of their target muscles (the constrictor pupillae and the ciliary muscles); therefore, they control the size of the pupil and the shape of the lens.

Pupillary Light Reflex

The pupillary light reflex is described in Chapter II. The parasympathetic axons that form part of the oculomotor nerve are the efferent, or motor limb of this reflex.

Accommodation Reflex

Accommodation is an adaptation of the visual apparatus of the eye for near vision (Figure III–8). It is accomplished by the following:

• An increase in the curvature of the lens. The suspensory ligament of the lens is attached to the lens periphery. At rest, the ligament maintains tension on the lens,

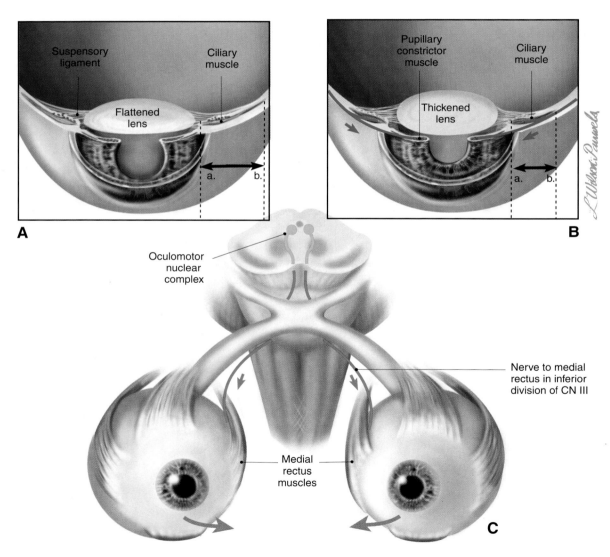

Figure III–8 *A,* Eye adjusted for distance vision: large pupil and relaxed ciliary muscle. *B,* In accommodation for near vision, the pupillary constrictor muscles contract resulting in a smaller pupil, and the ciliary muscles contract and the suspensory ligaments relax resulting in a thicker lens. *C,* The medial recti muscles contract causing the eyes to converge.

keeping it flat (see Figure III–8A). During accommodation, efferent axons from the Edinger-Westphal nucleus signal the ciliary muscle to contract (shortening the distance from "a" to "b"), which releases some of the tension of the suspensory ligament of the lens and allows the curvature of the lens to increase (see Figure III–8B).

- Pupillary constriction. The Edinger-Westphal nucleus also signals the sphincter-like pupillary constrictor muscle to contract. The resulting smaller pupil helps to sharpen the image on the retina (see Figure III–8B).
- Convergence of the eyes. The oculomotor nucleus sends signals to both medial rectus muscles, which cause them to contract. This, in turn, causes the eyes to converge (see Figure III–8C).

> The pathways that mediate these actions are not well understood, but it is clear that the reflex is initiated by the occipital (visual) cortex that sends signals to the oculomotor and Edinger-Westphal nuclei via the pretectal region. See Vergence System, Chapter 13.

CASE HISTORY GUIDING QUESTIONS

1. How did a posterior communicating artery aneurysm cause Werner's symptoms?

2. What is the significance of the light sensitivity Werner experienced in the two weeks preceding the subarachnoid hemorrhage?

3. When light was shone into Werner's right pupil, why did the left pupil constrict but not the right?

4. Where else along the course of cranial nerve III could damage occur?

5. How can a third nerve palsy caused by damage to the neuronal cell bodies in the oculomotor nucleus be differentiated from a third nerve palsy caused by damage to the axons within the nerve itself?

6. Why did Werner's right eye deviate downward and outward?

1. How did a posterior communicating artery aneurysm cause Werner's symptoms?

The third cranial nerve passes close to the posterior communicating artery (see Figure III–4). An aneurysm (an expansion of the diameter of a blood vessel) of the posterior communicating artery can compress cranial nerve III resulting in a lower motor neuron lesion (Figure III–9). In Werner's case, the aneurysm was compressing the right cranial nerve III causing his double vision and light sensitivity. Rupture of the aneurysm resulted in a subarachnoid hemorrhage, which caused his sudden, severe headache.

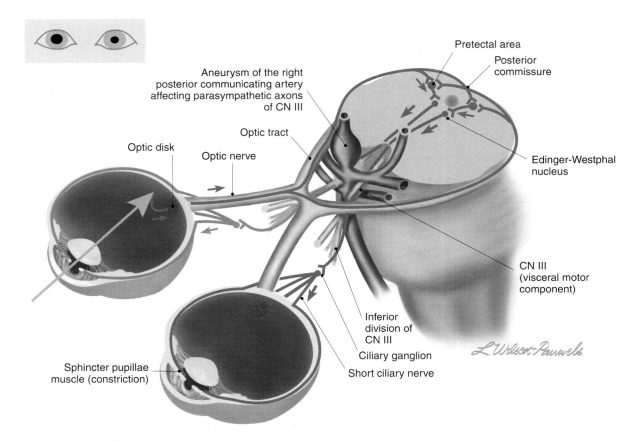

Figure III–9 Efferent pupillary defect. Light shone in Werner's right eye resulted in left pupillary constriction (indirect or consensual) with the absence of right pupillary constriction (direct) due to an aneurysm of the posterior communicating artery.

2. What is the significance of the light sensitivity Werner experienced in the two weeks preceding the subarachnoid hemorrhage?

The parasympathetic fibers responsible for constriction of the pupil in response to light lie on the surface of cranial nerve III (see Figure III–2 and Figure III–10). Initially, the aneurysm was small and, therefore, only the parasympathetic fibers were compromised. As a result, his right pupil could not constrict as well as usual in bright light, which caused his light sensitivity.

When the third nerve becomes ischemic, for example, in diabetes or stroke, the somatic motor axons in the center of the nerve are affected; however, the parasympatheic axons on the surface of the nerve are relatively spared. In this case, the patient has an oculomotor palsy with sparing of the pupillary light reflex—the opposite of Werner's early dysfunction.

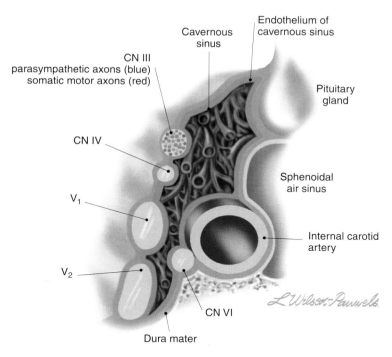

Figure III–10 Slice through the right cavernous sinus showing the relationship of cranial nerve III to other structures coursing through the sinus.

3. When light was shone into Werner's right pupil, why did the left pupil constrict but not the right?

The aneurysm of the posterior communicating artery compressed the right oculomotor nerve but did not affect the optic nerve. When light was shone into the right eye, the afferent (special sensory) limb of the pupillary light response was intact. Light shone into either pupil causes signals to be sent along the optic nerve, which bilaterally innervate the Edinger-Westphal nuclei. Visceral motor signals that arise from these nuclei are transmitted along the parasympathetic fibers in cranial nerve III. In Werner's case, these fibers are intact on the left side but damaged on the right. Therefore, the left pupil constricted in response to both direct and indirect stimulation, but the right pupil did not constrict in either case (see Figure III–9).

Compare Werner's *efferent* pupillary defect (see Figure III–9) with Meredith's *afferent* pupillary defect shown in Chapter II, Figure II–12.

4. Where else along the course of cranial nerve III could damage occur?

Cranial nerve III can be damaged anywhere from the nucleus in the midbrain to the muscles of innervation.

Cranial nerve III can be damaged at the following sites.

Nucleus of Cranial Nerve III

- Although rare, damage to cells in the nucleus of cranial nerve III may be due to trauma, ischemia, or demyelination within the midbrain.

Peripheral Axons

- Damage to axons in the subarachnoid space may be due to infection, tumor infiltration, or infarction (loss of blood supply, usually caused by diabetes or hypertension).
- Compression of axons may be due to aneurysms, most typically in the posterior communicating artery and sometimes in the basilar artery (see Figure III–9).
- Compression of axons may be caused by the uncus of the temporal lobe during cerebral herniation if there is raised intracranial pressure.
- Compression of axons in the cavernous sinus may be due to tumors, inflammation, infection, or thrombosis (other nerves that pass through the cavernous sinus [IV, V_1, V_2, VI] may also be involved) (see Figure III–10).
- Damage may be caused by trauma to the area where axons pass through the superior orbital fissure to enter the orbit.

5. How can a third nerve palsy caused by damage to the neuronal cell bodies in the oculomotor nucleus be differentiated from a third nerve palsy caused by damage to the axons within the nerve itself?

Because the oculomotor nucleus is close to the midline, it is extremely rare to have a unilateral nuclear lesion (Figure III–11A). To distinguish a nuclear lesion from an axonal lesion, a useful indictor is the behavior of the upper eyelid.

In a nuclear lesion, there is

- bilateral innervation of the levator palpebrae superioris muscle by the central subnucleus and, therefore, there is no ptosis;
- ipsilateral innervation of the medial rectus muscle by the lateral subnucleus and, therefore, ipsilateral weakness of adduction;
- ipsilateral innervation of the inferior rectus muscle by the lateral subnucleus and, therefore, ipsilateral weakness of downward gaze;
- contralateral innervation of the superior rectus muscle and, therefore, there is no weakness in upward gaze in the ipsilateral eye; and
- ipsilateral innervation of the pupil by the Edinger-Westphal nucleus resulting in an ipsilateral dilated unresponsive pupil.

In contrast, when the peripheral part of the third nerve is damaged (axonal damage), innervation of all target muscles is affected and there is ptosis and a dilated unresponsive pupil on the ipsilateral side (Figure III–11B). Both lesions described above are lower motor neuron lesions.

6. Why did Werner's right eye deviate downward and outward?

Werner has a lower motor neuron lesion of the right cranial nerve III (see Introduction for the general characteristics of a lower motor neuron lesion).

His symptoms include the following:

- strabismus (inability to direct both his eyes toward the same object) and consequent diplopia (double vision);

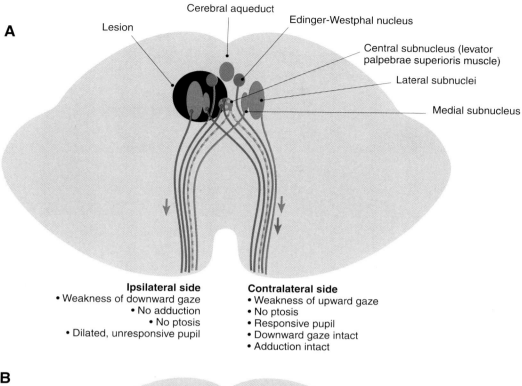

A

Cerebral aqueduct

Lesion

Edinger-Westphal nucleus

Central subnucleus (levator palpebrae superioris muscle)

Lateral subnuclei

Medial subnucleus

Ipsilateral side
- Weakness of downward gaze
- No adduction
- No ptosis
- Dilated, unresponsive pupil

Contralateral side
- Weakness of upward gaze
- No ptosis
- Responsive pupil
- Downward gaze intact
- Adduction intact

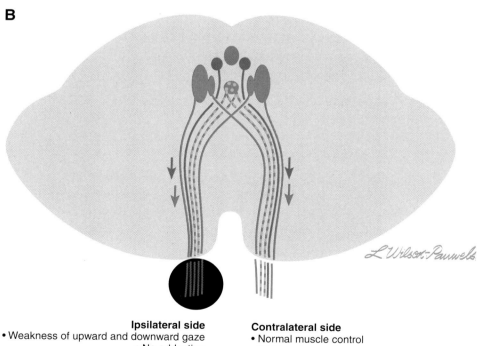

B

Ipsilateral side
- Weakness of upward and downward gaze
- No adduction
- Ptosis
- Dilated, unresponsive pupil

Contralateral side
- Normal muscle control
- Responsive pupil
- No ptosis

Figure III–11 *A*, Right unilateral nuclear lower motor neuron lesion of cranial nerve III. *B*, Right unilateral peripheral lower motor neuron lesion of cranial nerve III.

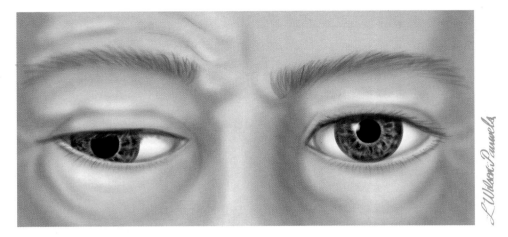

Figure III–12 Right third nerve palsy.

- right-sided ptosis (lid droop) due to inactivation of the levator palpebrae superioris muscle and the subsequent unopposed action of the orbicularis oculi muscle. Werner tries to compensate for ptosis by contracting his frontalis muscle to raise his eyebrow and attached lid;
- dilation of his right pupil due to decreased tone of the constrictor pupillae muscle;
- downward, abducted right eye postion due to the unopposed action of his right superior oblique and lateral rectus muscles; and
- inability to accommodate with his right eye.

This combination of symptoms is called a third nerve palsy (Figure III–12).

CLINICAL TESTING

Testing of cranial nerve III involves the assessment of

- eyelid position,
- pupillary response to light,
- extraocular eye movements, and
- accommodation.

(See also Cranial Nerves Examination on CD-ROM.)

Eyelid Position

Elevation of the eyelid results from activation of the levator palpebrae superioris muscle. Damage to cranial nerve III will result in ipsilateral or bilateral ptosis (drooping of the eyelid[s]). To assess the function of the muscle, ask the patient to look directly ahead and note the position of the edge of the upper eyelid relative to the iris. The eyelid should not droop over the pupil, and the eyelid position should be symmetric on both sides (Figure III–13).

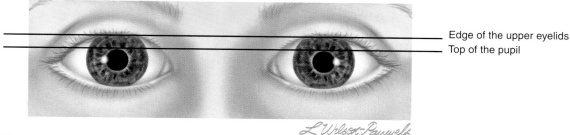

Edge of the upper eyelids
Top of the pupil

Figure III–13 Normal eyelid position.

Pupillary Response to Light

The afferent limb of the pupillary light reflex is carried by cranial nerve II—the optic nerve (Figure III–14). The efferent component of the pupillary light reflex is carried by parasympathetic fibers that travel on the surface of cranial nerve III (see Figure III–10). To assess the integrity of the reflex, a beam of focused light is shone directly into one pupil. In the normal reflex, light shone in the ipsilateral eye causes the ipsilateral pupil to constrict (direct light response). The contralateral pupil also constricts (indirect or consensual response) (see Figure III–14). If the afferent arm (cranial nerve II) is intact but the ipsilateral efferent pathway is damaged, the ipsilateral pupil will not constrict but the contralateral pupil will (see Figure III–9).

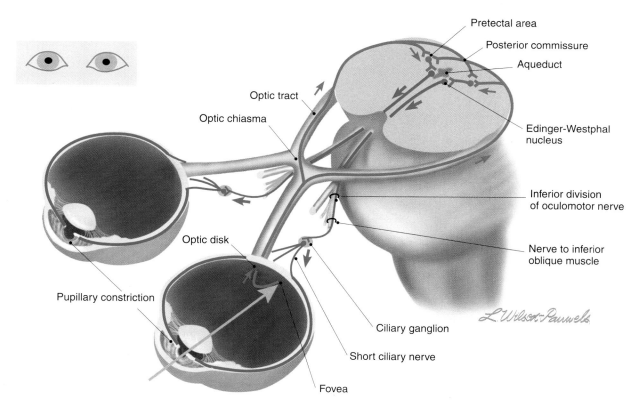

Pretectal area
Posterior commissure
Aqueduct
Optic tract
Optic chiasma
Edinger-Westphal nucleus
Inferior division of oculomotor nerve
Nerve to inferior oblique muscle
Optic disk
Pupillary constriction
Ciliary ganglion
Short ciliary nerve
Fovea

Figure III–14 Pupillary light reflex. Light shone in either eye (*left illustrated*) causes direct (ipsilateral) and indirect or consensual (contralateral) pupillary constriction.

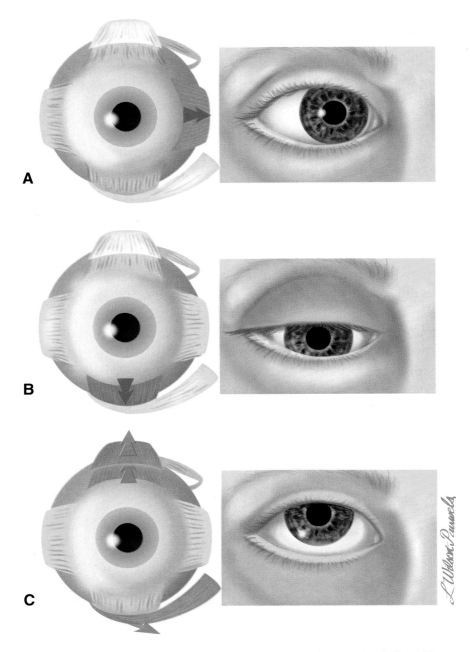

Figure III–15 Movements of the right eye and lids controlled by the muscles (colored) innervated by the oculomotor nerve (cranial nerve III). *A*, Adduction—medial rectus muscle (cranial nerve III). *B*, Downward gaze—inferior rectus muscle (cranial nerve III) aided by the superior oblique muscle (cranial nerve IV). The tendon of the inferior rectus muscle extends into the lower eyelid, pulling it down during downward gaze. *C*, Upward gaze—superior rectus aided by the inferior oblique muscle (cranial nerve III). The upper eyelid is raised by the levator palpebrae superioris muscle.

Extraocular Eye Movements

Cranial nerve III is tested in conjunction with cranial nerves IV and VI through assessment of extraocular eye movements (see Chapter 13). When testing the integrity of cranial nerve III, particular attention should be paid to adducting and vertical eye movements. If a lesion is present, eye adduction may be impaired because cranial nerve III innervates the medial rectus muscle (Figure III–15A). Cranial nerve III also innervates the inferior rectus, which controls part of downward gaze (Figure III–15B), and the superior rectus muscle and the inferior oblique muscle, which are responsible for upward gaze (Figure III–15C). Thus, if a lesion is present, vertical eye movements may also be impaired.

Accommodation

Accommodation allows the visual apparatus of the eye to focus on a near object. The observable events in accommodation are convergence and pupillary constriction of both eyes. Accommodation is tested by asking the patient to follow the examiner's finger as it is brought from a distance toward the patient's nose. As the examiner's finger approaches the patient's nose, the patient's eyes converge and his or her pupils constrict (Figure III–16).

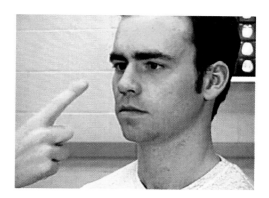

Figure III–16 Testing cranial nerve III for accommodation.

ADDITIONAL RESOURCES

Brodal A. Neurological anatomy in relation to clinical medicine. 3rd ed. New York: Oxford University Press; 1981. p. 532–77.

Glimcher PA. Eye movements. In: Zigmond MJ, Bloom FE, Landis SC, et al, editors. Fundamental neuroscience. San Diego: Academic Press; 1999. p. 993–1009.

Porter JD. Brainstem terminations of extraocular muscle primary sensory afferent neurons in the monkey. J Comp Neurol 1986;247:133–43.

IV Trochlear Nerve

*innervates
the superior
oblique muscle
of the eye*

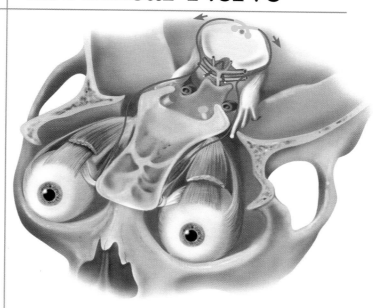

IV Trochlear Nerve

CASE HISTORY

Harpinder is a 53-year-old woman with long-standing diabetes and hypertension. She was out for an afternoon walk when she experienced the onset of headache behind her right eye. It was a continuous dull pain and, although not severe, caused her to cut her walk short. While walking home, she experienced intermittent double vision. Harpinder assumed that she was just tired and expected it to pass. After arriving home, as she began to prepare the evening dinner, she noticed that her double vision worsened when she was looking down at the chopping board, but it improved if she tilted her head to the left or if she looked up. Alarmed that something was wrong, Harpinder went to the hospital.

Initially, Harpinder was assessed by the resident. The resident found that Harpinder's eye movements were normal, and he could not account for her double vision. Review of the case with a staff neurologist gave some clues to her problem. Harpinder's pupils were equal in size and reactive to light, and there was no evidence of ptosis (upper eyelid droop). Harpinder was able to move her eyes fully through the horizontal planes. However, when the neurologist tested Harpinder's vertical eye movements, with her eyes abducted and adducted, he discovered that Harpinder could not look down with her right eye when it was adducted. Harpinder also noticed that she had double vision in this position and that the image from her right eye was superior and parallel to the image from her left eye. The neurologist diagnosed a right cranial nerve IV palsy and attributed it to infarction of the nerve due to diabetes.

ANATOMY OF THE TROCHLEAR NERVE

The trochlear nerve, the smallest of the cranial nerves, innervates only a single muscle in the orbit: the superior oblique muscle (Figure IV–1A). It has only a somatic motor component (Table IV–1). The cell bodies of the lower motor neurons constitute the trochlear nucleus, which is located in the tegmentum of the midbrain at the level of the inferior colliculus (Figure IV–1B). Like other somatic motor nuclei, the trochlear nucleus is close to the midline. Motor neurons from the trochlear nucleus innervate predominantly, if not exclusively, the contralateral superior oblique muscle. Axons arising from the trochlear nucleus course dorsally around the periaqueductal grey matter and cerebral aqueduct and cross the midline (Figure IV–1C). The crossed axons emerge from the dorsal aspect of the midbrain just caudal to the inferior colliculus to form the fourth cranial nerve. The nerve curves ventrally around the cerebral peduncle to pass between the posterior cerebral and superior cerebellar arteries lateral to the third cranial nerve. Cranial nerve IV runs anteriorly to pierce the dura at the angle between the free and attached borders of the tentorium cerebelli.

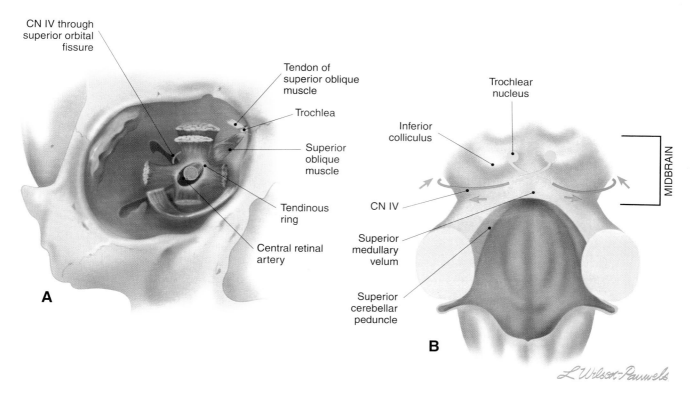

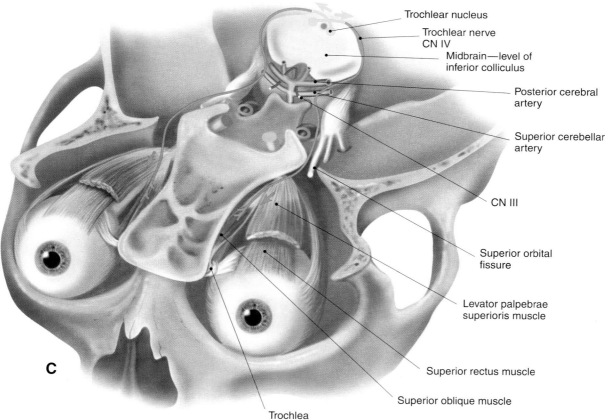

Figure IV–1 *A*, Apex of the right orbit illustrating the tendinous ring. *B*, Dorsal aspect of the brain stem. *C*, Somatic motor tract from the trochlear nucleus in the brain stem to the superior oblique muscle.

Table IV–1 Nerve Fiber Modality and Function of the Trochlear Nerve

Nerve Fiber Modality	Nucleus	Function
Somatic motor (efferent)	Trochlear	Innervation of the superior oblique muscle of the eye

Cranial nerve IV enters the cavernous sinus along with cranial nerves III, V_1, V_2, and VI. Within the cavernous sinus, the trochlear nerve is situated between nerves III and V_1 and lateral to the internal carotid artery (Figure IV–2). It leaves the cavernous sinus and enters the orbit through the superior orbital fissure, above the tendinous ring (see Figure IV–1A). The nerve then courses medially, close to the roof of the orbit, and runs diagonally above the levator palpebrae superioris muscle to reach its target, the superior oblique muscle. Here the nerve divides into three or more branches that enter the superior oblique muscle along its proximal third.

Eye Movements

The tendon of the superior oblique muscle loops through a "pulley" of fibrocartilage (the *trochlea*) in the connective tissue of the superior anteromedial corner of the orbit and then turns posterolateral to insert into the sclera in the superolateral posterior quadrant of the eye (Figure IV–3). Contraction of the muscle, therefore, pulls the posterolateral surface of the eyeball forward.

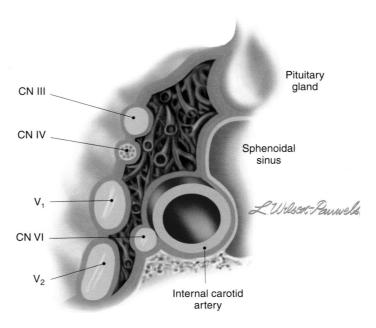

Figure IV–2 Slice through the right cavernous sinus showing the relationship of cranial nerve IV to other structures coursing through the sinus.

ADDUCTED POSITION

AT REST   IN ACTION

NEUTRAL POSITION

AT REST   IN ACTION

ABDUCTED POSITION

AT REST   IN ACTION

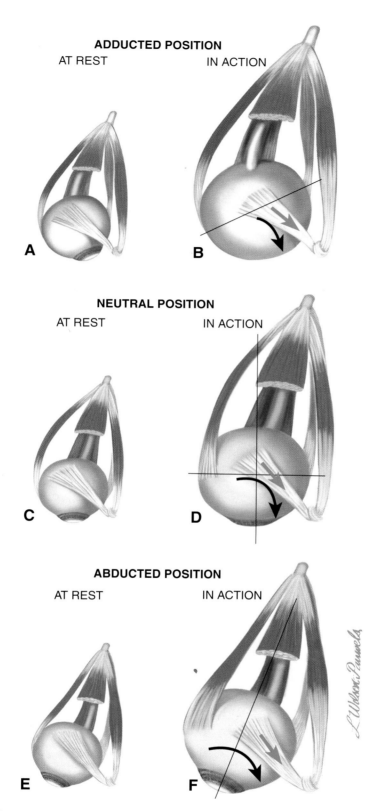

Figure IV–3 Movements of the right eye produced by the action of the superior oblique muscle in different eye positions (viewed from above). For rotation around axes, see Figure IV–4. *A,* At rest, adducted position. *B,* When the eye is adducted (toward the nose, rotation around the Y axis), the pull of the superior oblique muscle (*pink arrow*) causes downward movement of the cornea (*black arrow*). *C,* At rest, neutral position. *D,* When the eye is in a neutral position (looking straight ahead, rotation around both Y and Z axes), the pull of the superior oblique muscle (*pink arrow*) causes both downward movement of the cornea and intorsion (*black arrow*). *E,* At rest, abducted position. *F,* When the eye is abducted (away from the nose, rotation around the Z axis), the pull of the superior oblique muscle (*pink arrow*) causes intorsion (*black arrow*).

The actual movement caused by the superior oblique muscle depends on the initial position of the eye (Table IV–2 and Figure IV–4).

Table IV–2 Eye Movements Mediated by Cranial Nerve IV

Nerve	Muscle	Primary Action	Subsidiary Action
CN IV	Superior oblique	Downward gaze	Intorsion, abduction

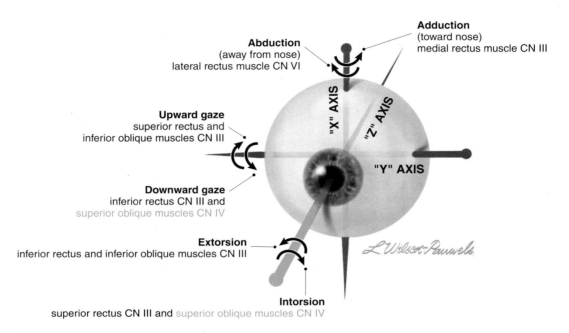

Figure IV–4 Right eye movements around the "X," "Y," and "Z" axes. Movements driven by cranial nerve IV are highlighted in pink.

CASE HISTORY GUIDING QUESTIONS

1. Why did Harpinder have double vision?

2. Why did Harpinder's double vision improve when she tilted her head to the left?

3. What other lesions could affect the trochlear nerve?

4. Why did the resident not identify Harpinder's eye movement problem?

1. Why did Harpinder have double vision?

Harpinder's right superior oblique muscle is not functioning. As a result, its antagonist muscle, the inferior oblique, extorts and slightly elevates her right eye (Figure IV–5). Consequently, the visual fields are projected onto different areas of Harpinder's right and left retinae and she perceives two distinct images.

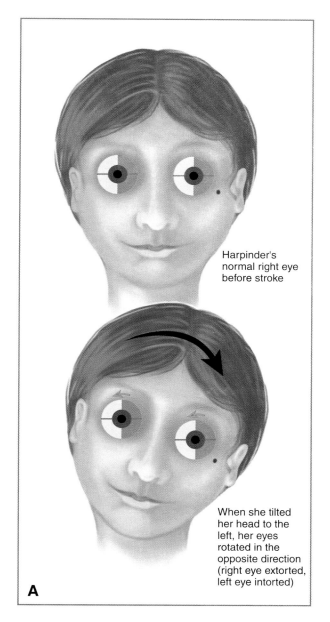

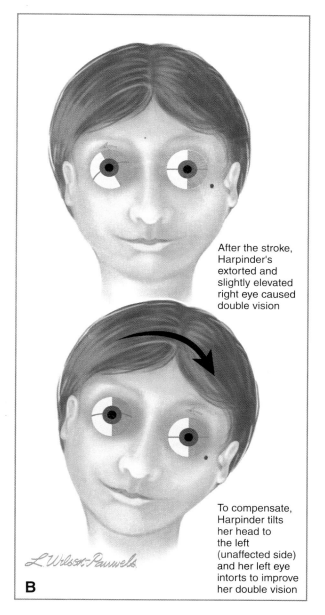

Figure IV–5 Ocular rotation. *A*, Before Harpinder's stroke; *B*, after Harpinder's stroke.

2. Why did Harpinder's double vision improve when she tilted her head to the left?

Normally, as the head tilts from side to side, the eyes rotate in the opposite direction (see Figure IV–5A). Because Harpinder's right superior oblique muscle was paralysed, her right eye was extorted and slightly elevated (see Figure IV–5B, upper figure). When she tilted her head to the left, her normal left eye intorted and her double vision improved (see Figure IV–5B, lower figure).

3. What other lesions could affect the trochlear nerve?

The trochlear nerve can be damaged anywhere from its nucleus in the midbrain to its termination in the orbit. The intramedullary axons can be damaged in the midbrain by infarction, tumor, or demyelination. The nerve can be damaged in the subarachnoid space by trauma, tumor, and meningitis. Within the cavernous sinus, aneurysm of the internal carotid artery, cavernous sinus thrombosis, tumors, and inflammation can all damage cranial nerve IV. The nerve can also be affected by ischemia; this is most commonly seen in patients with diabetes or hypertension.

4. Why did the resident not identify Harpinder's eye movement problem?

The superior oblique muscle has two major actions: intorsion of the eye (ie, rotation around the anteroposterior axis) and downward gaze (see Figure IV–4). Since the eye is radially symmetric, rotation about the anteroposterior axis is very difficult to detect (but watching the movement of the conjunctival vessels is sometimes helpful). A better test of the superior oblique muscle is to examine downward gaze when the eye is adducted (Figure IV–6). The resident did not test Harpinder's vertical eye movements with her right eye adducted and, thus, missed the abnormality.

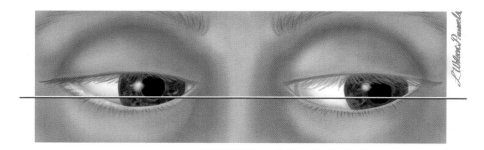

Figure IV–6 Harpinder is unable to move her right eye downward.

CLINICAL TESTING

Cranial nerve IV is tested in conjunction with cranial nerves III and VI through the assessment of eye movements (see Chapter 13). (See also Cranial Nerves Examination on CD-ROM.)

ADDITIONAL RESOURCES

Brodal A. Neurological anatomy in relation to clinical medicine. 3rd ed. New York: Oxford University Press; 1981. p. 532–77.

Glimcher PA. Eye movements. In: Zigmond MJ, Bloom FE, Landis SC, et al, editors. Fundamental neuroscience. San Diego: Academic Press; 1999. p. 993–1009.

Porter JD. Brainstem terminations of extraocular muscle primary sensory afferent neurons in the monkey. J Comp Neurol 1986;247:133–43.

Spencer RF, McNeer KW. The periphery: extraocular muscles and motor neurons. In: Carpenter RHS, editor. Eye movements. Boca Raton: CRC Press Inc.; 1991. p. 175–99.

V | Trigeminal Nerve

*carries
general sensation
from the
face and head
and innervates
the muscles
of mastication*

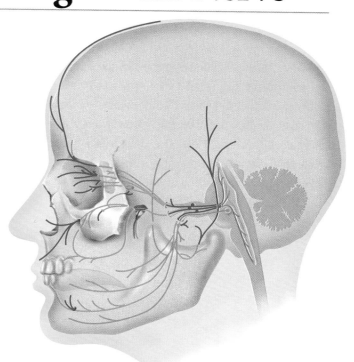

V Trigeminal Nerve

CASE HISTORY

For the last few months, Mary, a 55-year-old professor, has been experiencing sudden attacks of extreme but short-lived pain on the left side of her face. She described the pain as "hornet stings" shooting through her jaw. The pain could be elicited by brushing her teeth, stroking the left side of her face, or talking. She initially thought her problem was related to her teeth and went to the dentist. Her dentist was unable to find anything wrong with her teeth and suggested that she see her family doctor.

When she saw her family doctor, Mary explained that the pain was most frequent when she was lecturing in class and had become so frequent and severe that she was finding it difficult to continue teaching. The doctor did a neurologic examination and found that her cranial nerves were functioning normally. He suggested that her pain was probably due to hyperexcitablilty of her fifth cranial nerve (the trigeminal nerve) and diagnosed trigeminal neuralgia. To treat this condition he prescribed carbamazepine. Initially, Mary's symptoms improved; however, months later they returned and, despite trials with other anticonvulsants, the pain persisted. Because Mary was not improving, her doctor ordered magnetic resonance imaging (MRI) and referred her to a neurosurgeon for consideration of surgical treatment of her condition.

ANATOMY OF THE TRIGEMINAL NERVE

Embryologically, the trigeminal nerve is the nerve of the first branchial arch. The name trigeminal (literally, three twins) refers to the fact that the fifth cranial nerve has three major divisions: the *ophthalmic* (V_1), *maxillary* (V_2), and *mandibular* (V_3) divisions (Figures V–1 and V–2). It is the major sensory nerve of the face and innervates several muscles that are listed in Table V–1.

The trigeminal nerve emerges on the midlateral surface of the pons as a large sensory root and a smaller motor root. Its sensory ganglion (the semilunar or trigeminal or gasserian ganglion) sits in a depression called the trigeminal cave (Meckel's cave), in the floor of the middle cranial fossa. Sensory axons at the distal aspect of the ganglion form the three major divisions (V_1, V_2, and V_3). The motor axons travel with the mandibular division (V_3).

Table V–1 Nerve Fiber Modality and Function of the Trigeminal Nerve

Nerve Fiber Modality	Nucleus	Function
General sensory (afferent)	Spinal trigeminal	Pain and temperature Simple touch All general sensory modalities from the face and anterior scalp as far as the apex of the head, conjunctiva, bulb of the eye, mucous membranes of paranasal sinuses, and nasal and oral cavities including tongue and teeth, part of the external aspect of the tympanic membrane, and from the meninges of the anterior and middle cranial fossae*
	Pontine trigeminal Mesencephalic	Discriminative touch Proprioception Vibration sense
Branchial motor (efferent)	Motor (masticator)	Innervation of the muscles of mastication, (ie, masseter, temporalis, medial and lateral pterygoid muscles, plus tensores tympani, tensores veli palatini, mylohyoid, and anterior belly of the digastric muscles)

*Meninges of the posterior cranial fossa receive their sensory innervation from the upper few cervical nerves.

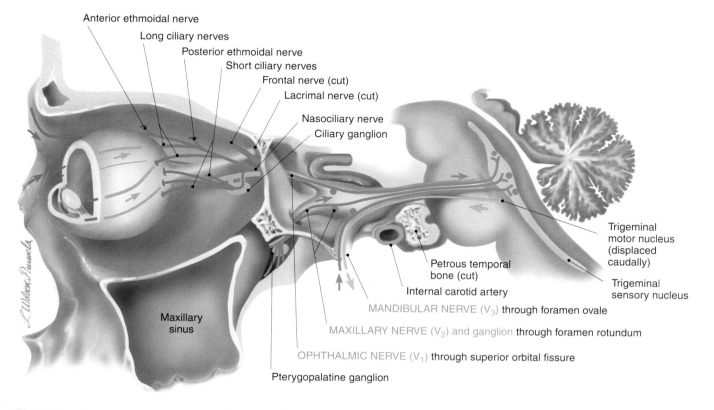

Figure V–1 Parasagittal section through the skull showing the trigeminal ganglion and its three major divisions. The long and short ciliary nerves are featured. The motor (masticator) nucleus has been displaced caudally for illustrative purposes. It lies medial to the chief sensory nucleus.

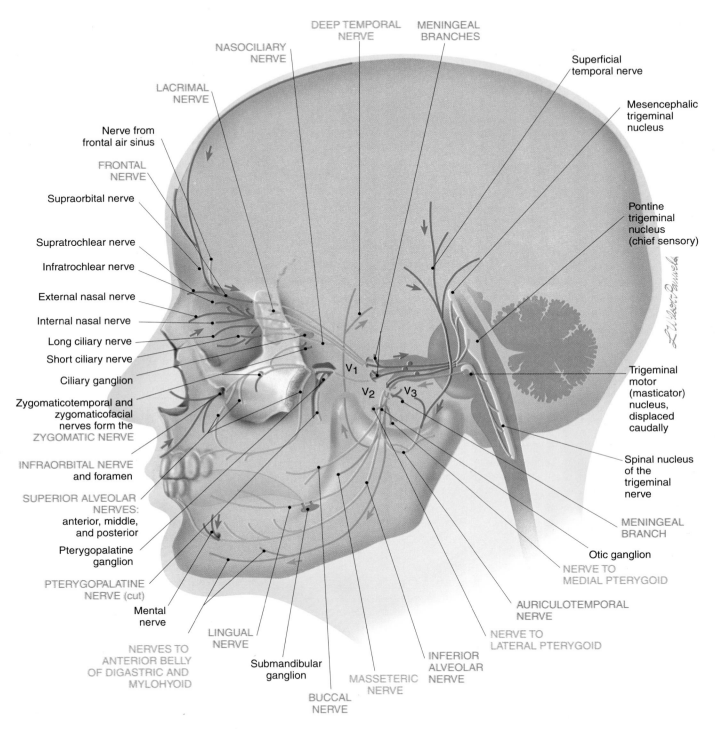

DEEP TEMPORAL NERVE

MENINGEAL BRANCHES

NASOCILIARY NERVE

Superficial temporal nerve

LACRIMAL NERVE

Mesencephalic trigeminal nucleus

Nerve from frontal air sinus

FRONTAL NERVE

Supraorbital nerve

Pontine trigeminal nucleus (chief sensory)

Supratrochlear nerve

Infratrochlear nerve

External nasal nerve

Internal nasal nerve

Long ciliary nerve

Short ciliary nerve

Ciliary ganglion

Trigeminal motor (masticator) nucleus, displaced caudally

Zygomaticotemporal and zygomaticofacial nerves form the ZYGOMATIC NERVE

Spinal nucleus of the trigeminal nerve

INFRAORBITAL NERVE and foramen

SUPERIOR ALVEOLAR NERVES: anterior, middle, and posterior

MENINGEAL BRANCH

Pterygopalatine ganglion

Otic ganglion

PTERYGOPALATINE NERVE (cut)

NERVE TO MEDIAL PTERYGOID

Mental nerve

AURICULOTEMPORAL NERVE

LINGUAL NERVE

NERVE TO LATERAL PTERYGOID

NERVES TO ANTERIOR BELLY OF DIGASTRIC AND MYLOHYOID

Submandibular ganglion

INFERIOR ALVEOLAR NERVE

MASSETERIC NERVE

BUCCAL NERVE

V₁ V₂ V₃

Figure V–2 Overview of the trigeminal nerve.

GENERAL SENSORY (AFFERENT) COMPONENT

Ophthalmic Division (V₁)

The ophthalmic division has three major branches (Table V–2): the frontal, lacrimal, and nasociliary nerves (Figures V–3 and V–4). The *frontal nerve* is formed by the supraorbital nerve from the forehead and scalp and the supratrochlear nerve from the bridge of the nose, medial part of the upper eyelid, and medial forehead. A small sensory twig from the frontal air sinus joins the frontal nerve near the anterior part of the orbit.

The *lacrimal nerve* carries sensory information from the lateral part of the upper eyelid, conjunctiva, and lacrimal gland. It runs posteriorly near the roof of the orbit to join the frontal and nasociliary nerves at the superior orbital fissure. Secretomotor fibers to the lacrimal gland from cranial nerve VII (facial), may travel briefly with the lacrimal nerve in its peripheral portion.

The *nasociliary nerve* is formed by the convergence of several terminal branches. These are the infratrochlear nerve from the skin of the medial part of the eyelid and side of the nose, the external nasal nerve from the skin of the ala and apex of the nose, the internal nasal nerve from the anterior part of the nasal septum and lateral wall of the nasal cavity, the anterior and posterior ethmoidal nerves from the ethmoidal air sinuses, and the long and short ciliary nerves from the bulb of the eye.

The ophthalmic division leaves the orbit through the superior orbital fissure, passes through the cavernous sinus, and enters the trigeminal ganglion. Here it is joined by a meningeal branch from the tentorium cerebelli.

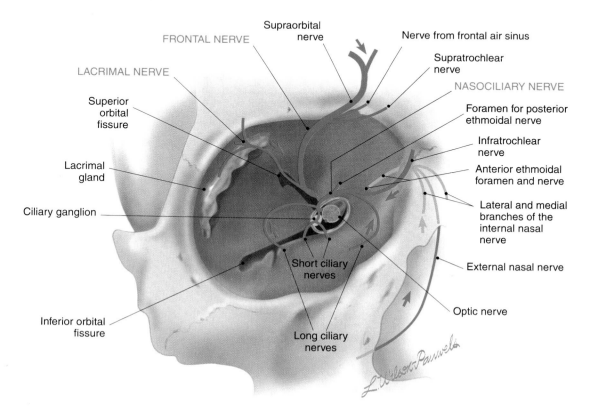

Figure V–3 Apex of right orbit illustrating branches of the ophthalmic division (V₁).

Table V–2 Branches of the Trigeminal Nerve

Division	General Sensory	Branchial Motor

Ophthalmic (V₁)	Lacrimal
	Frontal
	  Supratrochlear
	  Supraorbital
	    Nerve from frontal air sinus
	Nasociliary
	  Long and short ciliary
	  Infratrochlear
	  Ethmoidal
	    Anterior
	      Internal nasal
	        (medial and lateral)
	      External nasal
	    Posterior
	Meningeal branch
	  (from the tentorium cerebelli)	

Maxillary (V₂)	Zygomatic
	  Zygomaticotemporal
	  Zygomaticofacial
	Infraorbital
	  External nasal
	  Superior labial
	Superior alveolar
	    Posterior
	    Middle
	    Anterior
	Pterygopalatine
	  Orbital
	  Greater and lesser palatine
	  Posterior superior nasal
	  Pharyngeal
	Meningeal
	  (from the middle and anterior cranial fossae)	

Mandibular (V₃)	Buccal
	Lingual
	Inferior alveolar
	  Dental
	  Incisive
	  Mental
	Auriculotemporal
	  Anterior auricular
	  To external acoustic meatus
	  To temporomandibular joint
	  Superficial temporal
	Meningeal (spinosus)
	  (from the middle and anterior cranial fossae)
		Medial pterygoid
		  To tensor veli palatini
		  To tensor tympani
		Lateral pterygoid
		Masseteric
		Deep temporal
		To anterior belly of digastric
		To mylohyoid

The sensory components of the short ciliary nerves pass through the ciliary ganglion without synapsing. Proprioceptive sensory axons from the extraocular muscles travel initially with cranial nerves III, IV, and VI but leave them to join the ophthalmic division of the trigeminal nerve as it courses posteriorly through the cavernous sinus.

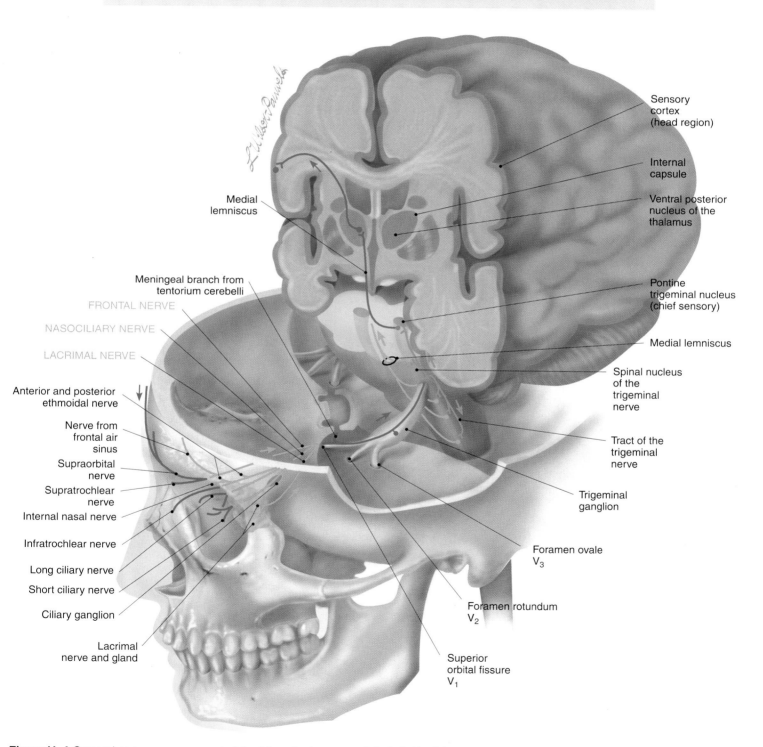

Figure V–4 General sensory component of the trigeminal nerve, ophthalmic V_1 division.

Maxillary Division (V₂)

The maxillary division is formed by the zygomatic, infraorbital, superior alveolar, and palatine nerves (Figures V–5 and V–6).

The *zygomatic nerve* has two major branches. Sensory processes from the prominence of the cheek converge to form the zygomaticofacial nerve. This nerve pierces the frontal process of the zygomatic bone and enters the orbit through its lateral wall. It turns posteriorly to join with the zygomaticotemporal nerve. Sensory processes from the side of the forehead converge to form the zygomaticotemporal nerve, which pierces the posterior aspect of the frontal process of the zygomatic bone, and traverses the lateral wall of the orbit to join with the zygomaticofacial nerve forming the zygomatic nerve. The zygomatic nerve courses posteriorly along the floor of the orbit to join with the maxillary nerve close to the inferior orbital fissure.

> Within the orbit, the zygomatic nerve travels briefly with postganglionic (parasympathetic) fibers from cranial nerve VII that are en route to the lacrimal gland (see Chapter VII, Figure VII–10).

The *infraorbital nerve* is formed by cutaneous branches from the upper lip, medial cheek, and side of the nose. It passes through the infraorbital foramen of the maxilla and travels posteriorly through the infraorbital canal where it is joined by anterior branches of the superior alveolar nerve. This combined trunk emerges on the floor of the orbit and becomes the maxillary nerve. The maxillary nerve continues posteriorly and is joined by the middle and posterior branches of the superior alveolar nerves and by the palatine nerves. The combined trunk, the maxillary division, enters the cranium through the foramen rotundum.

The *superior alveolar nerves* (anterior, middle, and posterior) carry sensory input, mainly pain, from the upper teeth.

The *palatine nerves* (see Figure V–6) (greater and lesser) originate in the hard and soft palates, respectively, and ascend toward the maxillary nerve through the pterygopalatine canal. En route, the palatine nerves are joined by a pharyngeal branch from the nasopharynx and by nasal branches from the posterior nasal cavity, including one particularly long branch, the *nasopalatine nerve*.

Small meningeal branches from the dura of the anterior and middle cranial fossae join the maxillary division as it enters the trigeminal ganglion (see Figure V–5).

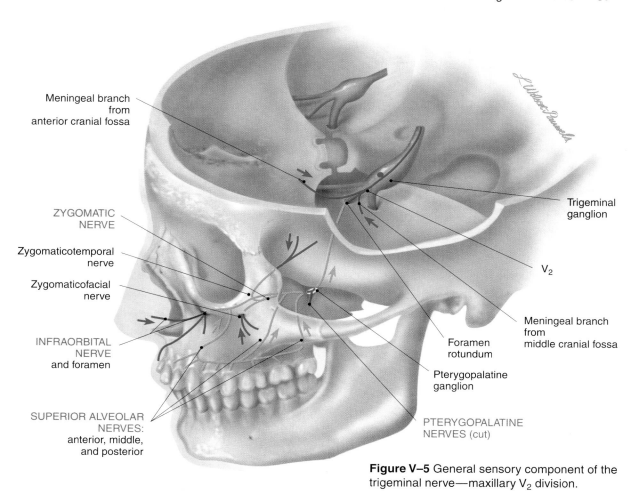

Meningeal branch from anterior cranial fossa

ZYGOMATIC NERVE

Zygomaticotemporal nerve

Zygomaticofacial nerve

INFRAORBITAL NERVE and foramen

SUPERIOR ALVEOLAR NERVES: anterior, middle, and posterior

Trigeminal ganglion

V₂

Meningeal branch from middle cranial fossa

Foramen rotundum

Pterygopalatine ganglion

PTERYGOPALATINE NERVES (cut)

Figure V–5 General sensory component of the trigeminal nerve—maxillary V_2 division.

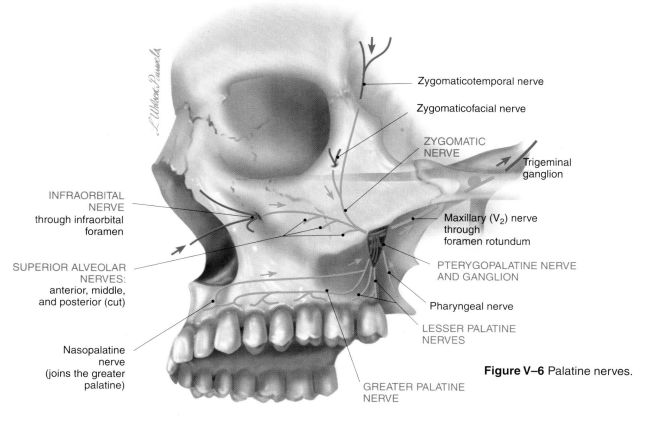

INFRAORBITAL NERVE through infraorbital foramen

SUPERIOR ALVEOLAR NERVES: anterior, middle, and posterior (cut)

Nasopalatine nerve (joins the greater palatine)

Zygomaticotemporal nerve

Zygomaticofacial nerve

ZYGOMATIC NERVE

Trigeminal ganglion

Maxillary (V_2) nerve through foramen rotundum

PTERYGOPALATINE NERVE AND GANGLION

Pharyngeal nerve

LESSER PALATINE NERVES

GREATER PALATINE NERVE

Figure V–6 Palatine nerves.

Mandibular Division (V₃)

The sensory component of V_3 is formed by the buccal, lingual, inferior alveolar, and auriculotemporal nerves (Figure V–7).

The *buccal nerve* (not to be confused with the nerve to buccinator, a motor branch of cranial nerve VII) carries sensory information from the buccal (cheek) region including the mucous membrane of the mouth and gums. The *buccal nerve* courses posteriorly in the cheek deep to the masseter muscle and pierces the lateral pterygoid muscle to join the main trunk of the mandibular nerve.

The *lingual* and *inferior alveolar nerves* carry general sensation from the entire lower jaw including the teeth, gums, and anterior two-thirds of the tongue.

Sensory axons from the tongue (anterior two-thirds) converge to form the lingual nerve, which runs posteriorly along the side of the tongue. At the back of the tongue, the lingual nerve curves upward to join the main trunk of the mandibular nerve deep to the lateral pterygoid muscle.

Sensory nerves from the chin and lower lip converge to form the mental nerve, which enters the mandible through the mental foramen to run in the mandibular canal. Within the canal, dental branches from the lower teeth join with the mental nerve to form the *inferior alveolar nerve*. This nerve continues posteriorly and exits from the mandibular canal through the mandibular foramen to join the main trunk of the mandibular division along with the lingual nerve.

The *auriculotemporal nerve*, which runs with the superficial temporal artery, carries sensation from the side of the head and scalp. Two main branches, the anterior and posterior auriculotemporal nerves and their tributaries, converge into a single trunk just anterior to the ear. Here they are joined by twigs from the external auditory meatus, the external surface of the tympanic membrane, and the temporomandibular joint. The nerve courses deep to the lateral pterygoid muscle and the neck of the mandible, splits to encircle the middle meningeal artery, and then joins the main trunk of the mandibular nerve. The entire mandibular division enters the cranium through the foramen ovale.

Sensation from the meninges of the anterior and middle cranial fossae is carried by the meningeal branch of the mandibular nerve. Two major meningeal trunks that travel with the middle meningeal artery converge into a single nerve, the nervus spinosus, which leaves the skull through the foramen spinosum. This nerve joins the main trunk of the mandibular nerve prior to returning to the cranial cavity through the foramen ovale.

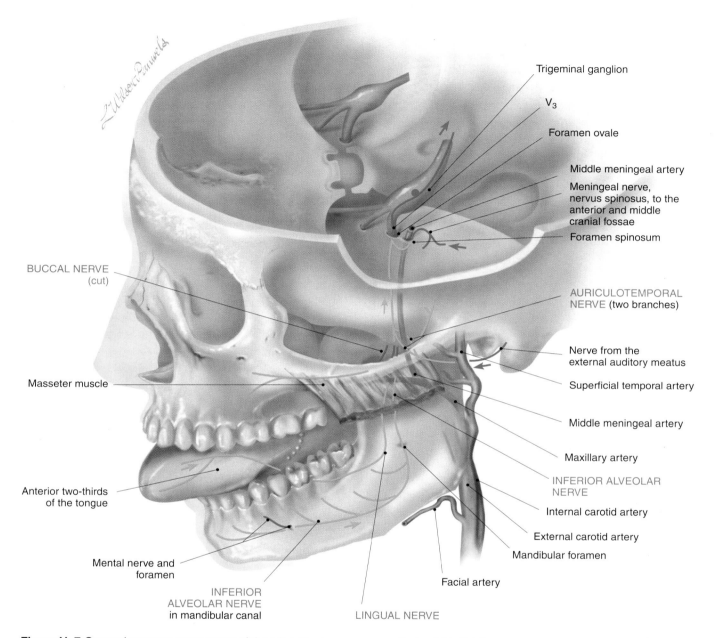

Trigeminal ganglion

V₃

Foramen ovale

Middle meningeal artery

Meningeal nerve, nervus spinosus, to the anterior and middle cranial fossae

Foramen spinosum

BUCCAL NERVE (cut)

AURICULOTEMPORAL NERVE (two branches)

Nerve from the external auditory meatus

Superficial temporal artery

Middle meningeal artery

Masseter muscle

Maxillary artery

INFERIOR ALVEOLAR NERVE

Anterior two-thirds of the tongue

Internal carotid artery

External carotid artery

Mandibular foramen

Mental nerve and foramen

Facial artery

INFERIOR ALVEOLAR NERVE in mandibular canal

LINGUAL NERVE

Figure V–7 General sensory component of the trigeminal nerve—mandibular (V₃) division.

Central Sensory Nuclei

All three divisions of the trigeminal nerve, ophthalmic, maxillary, and mandibular, join together at the trigeminal ganglion where most of the sensory nerve cell bodies reside. Central processes of these neurons constitute the sensory root of the trigeminal nerve, which enters the pons at its midlateral point. The axons terminate by synapsing with second-order sensory neurons in the appropriate region of the trigeminal nucleus.

The trigeminal nucleus (sensory nucleus of the trigeminal nerve) is the largest of the cranial nerve nuclei. It extends caudally from the midbrain into the spinal cord as far as the second cervical segment where it becomes continuous with the dorsal horn of the spinal cord (Figure V–8). Within the medulla it creates a lateral elevation—the tuberculum cinereum. It has three subnuclei: the mesencephalic nucleus, the pontine trigeminal (chief sensory) nucleus, and the spinal nucleus of the trigeminal nerve (Figures V–8 and V–9).

> The pontine trigeminal nucleus is known by a wide variety of names including the main, principal, chief, or superior trigeminal nucleus. In this text, we have chosen to use "pontine" to indicate its location, thereby maintaining consistency with the names of the other two subnuclei.

The mesencephalic trigeminal nucleus consists of a thin column of primary sensory neurons. Their peripheral processes, which travel with the motor nerves, carry proprioceptive information from the muscles of mastication. Their central processes project mainly to the motor nucleus of cranial nerve V (masticator nucleus) to provide for reflex control of the bite.

The pontine trigeminal nucleus is a large group of secondary sensory neurons located in the pons near the point of entry of the nerve. It is concerned primarily with discriminative touch sensation from the face.

The nucleus of the spinal trigeminal nerve, or spinal trigeminal nucleus, is a long column of cells extending from the pontine trigeminal nucleus caudally into the spinal cord where it merges with the dorsal gray matter of the spinal cord (Figure V–10). This subnucleus, especially its caudal portion, is concerned primarily with the perception of pain and temperature, although tactile information is projected to this subnucleus as well as to the pontine trigeminal nucleus. Axons of trigeminal nucleus neurons project to the contralateral sensory cortex via the thalamus, as detailed below.

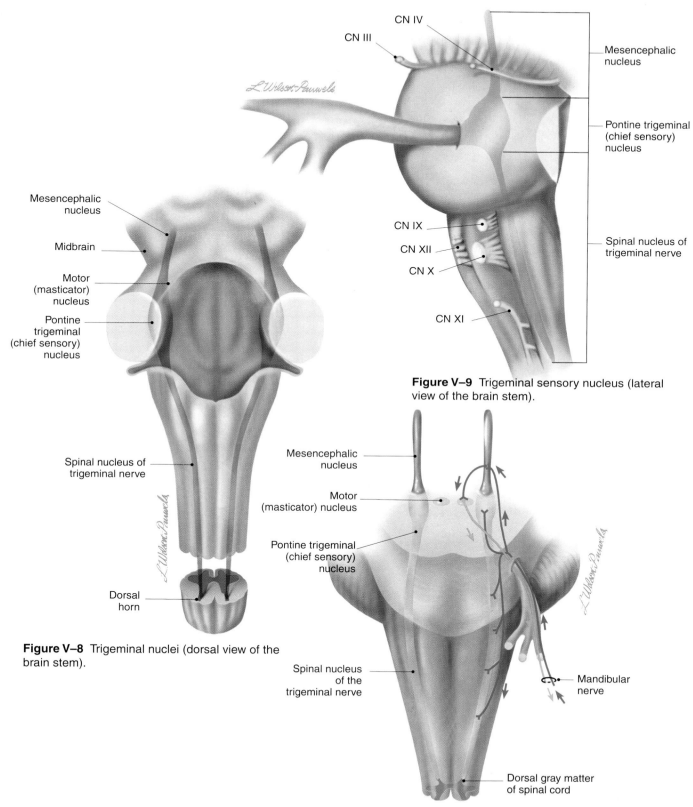

CN IV

CN III

Mesencephalic
nucleus

Pontine trigeminal
(chief sensory)
nucleus

CN IX

CN XII

CN X

Spinal nucleus of
trigeminal nerve

CN XI

Figure V–9 Trigeminal sensory nucleus (lateral
view of the brain stem).

Mesencephalic
nucleus

Midbrain

Motor
(masticator)
nucleus

Pontine
trigeminal
(chief sensory)
nucleus

Spinal nucleus of
trigeminal nerve

Dorsal
horn

Figure V–8 Trigeminal nuclei (dorsal view of the
brain stem).

Mesencephalic
nucleus

Motor
(masticator) nucleus

Pontine trigeminal
(chief sensory)
nucleus

Spinal nucleus
of the
trigeminal nerve

Mandibular
nerve

Dorsal gray matter
of spinal cord

Figure V–10 Trigeminal nucleus showing
sensory/motor reflex (ventral view of the brain stem).

CENTRAL PATHWAYS

There are two major sensory pathways that carry sensations from the face and sinuses to the cerebrum: the discriminative touch pathway (Figure V–11) and the pain and temperature pathway (Figure V–12).

Discriminative Touch Pathway

The discriminative touch pathway carries the sensory modalities of two-point discrimination: vibration sensation and proprioception. In terms of evolution, this pathway is a recent addition to the nervous system and is highly developed in primates.

Like most sensory pathways, the discriminative touch pathway includes three principal neurons.

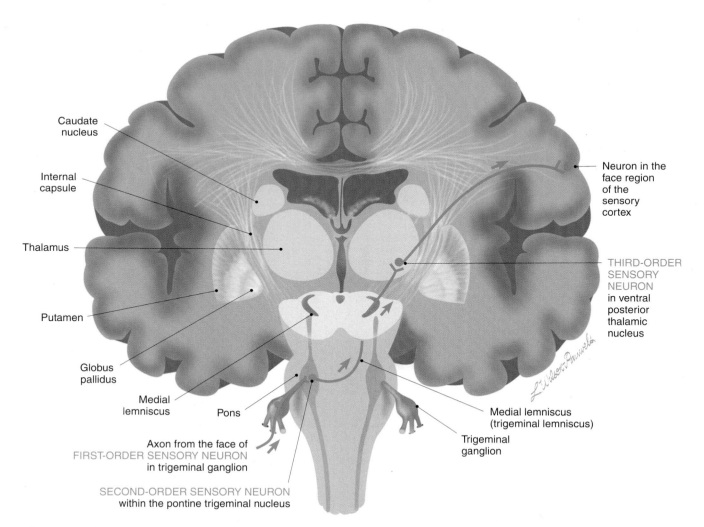

Figure V–11 The discriminative touch pathway from the head (see Clinical Testing).

1. The *first-order sensory neurons* carry information from a specific region of the face or meninges to the pontine trigeminal nucleus.

2. The pontine trigeminal nucleus is composed of cell bodies of *second-order sensory neurons*. Their axons leave this nucleus centrally, cross the midline, and join the medial lemniscus en route to the thalamus where they terminate within the ventral posterior thalamic nucleus.

3. Cell bodies of the *third-order sensory neurons* reside in the thalamus. Their axons leave the thalamus and travel through the posterior limb of the internal capsule and corona radiata to terminate in the appropriate region of the primary sensory cortex, where sensory signals are consciously perceived.

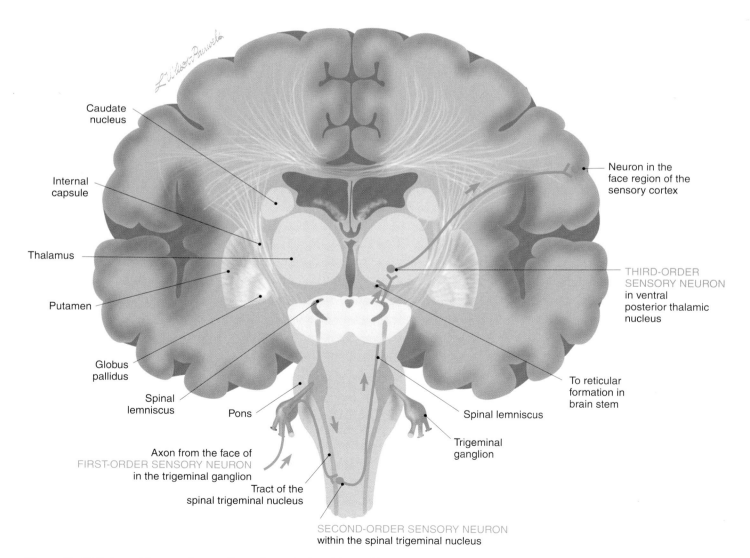

Figure V–12 Pain and temperature pathway from the head (see Clinical Testing).

Pain and Temperature Pathway

Pain and temperature sensation is carried by a much more primitive, widespread pathway than discriminative touch. In addition to the objective localization of pain sensation, the central pathways provide for activation of the limbic system and the activation of the fight or flight response that may be an appropriate response to pain. The trigeminal pain and temperature pathway also includes three principal neurons (see Figure V–12).

1. The *primary* or *first-order neuron* carries impulses from the periphery to the central nervous system. The central processes enter the pons along with the central processes of the discriminative touch neurons. Once they have entered the brain stem, they turn caudally and descend within the brain stem forming the tract of the spinal trigeminal nucleus before terminating within the appropriate parts of the nucleus.

2. Cell bodies of the *second-order sensory neuron* form the spinal trigeminal nucleus. Their axons cross the midline and join the spinal lemniscus en route to the thalamus where they terminate within the intralaminar and ventral posterior thalamic nuclei medial to the discriminative touch neurons. These axons also send collateral branches to the reticular formation in the brain stem, providing for arousal and visceral responses to pain.

3. Axons of *third-order (thalamic) neurons* project to the appropriate region of the sensory cortex where the sensory signals are consciously perceived.

Light or simple touch is poorly localized and is probably carried by both the discriminative touch and pain and temperature pathways.

In both discriminative touch and pain and temperature pathways, a small number of second-order sensory axons representing the mouth and perioral region ascends ipsilaterally to the ventral posterior nucleus of the thalamus providing for a degree of bilateral representation of the face within the sensory cortex.

BRANCHIAL MOTOR (EFFERENT) COMPONENT

Central Motor Nuclei: Innervation of the Masticator Nucleus

The trigeminal motor (masticator) nuclei are located in the tegmentum of the pons, medial to the pontine trigeminal nuclei (Figure V–13). They innervate the muscles of mastication (ie, masseters, temporales, medial and lateral pterygoid muscles, plus tensores tympani, tensores veli palatini, mylohyoid muscles, and anterior bellies of the digastric muscles).

In humans, jaw movements have two functions: a primitive function in masticating food and an important function in articulating speech sounds. Since chewing is primarily a reflex activity in response to sensory signals from the mouth, the

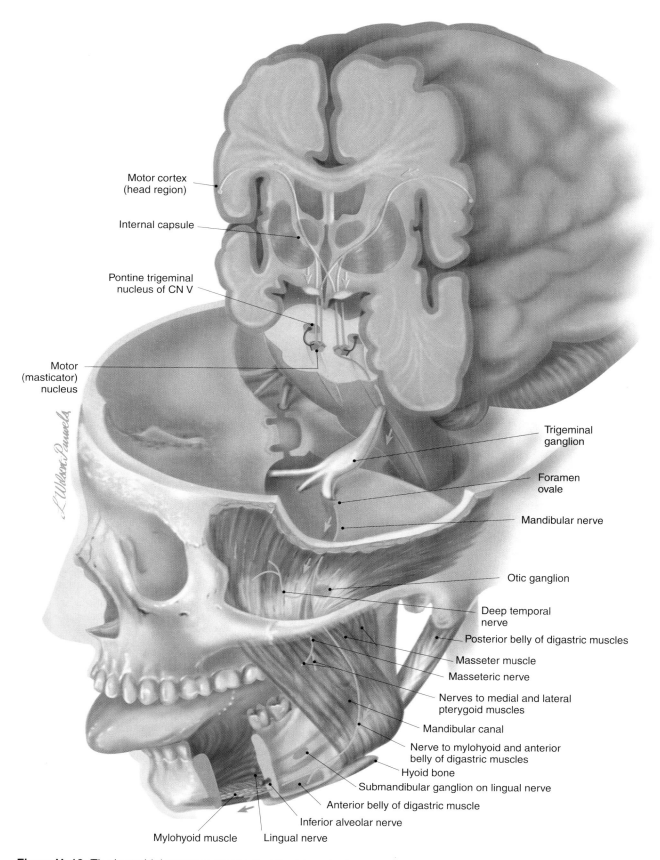

Motor cortex
(head region)

Internal capsule

Pontine trigeminal
nucleus of CN V

Motor
(masticator)
nucleus

Trigeminal
ganglion

Foramen
ovale

Mandibular nerve

Otic ganglion

Deep temporal
nerve

Posterior belly of digastric muscles

Masseter muscle

Masseteric nerve

Nerves to medial and lateral
pterygoid muscles

Mandibular canal

Nerve to mylohyoid and anterior
belly of digastric muscles

Hyoid bone

Submandibular ganglion on lingual nerve

Anterior belly of digastric muscle

Inferior alveolar nerve

Mylohyoid muscle   Lingual nerve

Figure V–13 The branchial motor component of the trigeminal nerve.

masticator nucleus receives its major inputs from sensory branches of the trigeminal nerve, both directly and via the pontine reticular formation. In addition, it receives signals from both cerebral hemispheres that mediate the jaw movements involved in speech and voluntary chewing.

Input from the vestibulocochlear nerve activates the part of the nucleus that innervates the tensor tympani, so that the tension of the tympanic membrane (ear drum) can be adjusted for sound intensity (see Chapter VIII, Figure VIII–1).

Peripheral Nerves

The motor nerves to the muscles of mastication travel with the mandibular division of the trigeminal nerve (Figures V–13 and V–14). Axons from the masticator nucleus (lower motor neurons) course laterally through the pons to exit as the motor root on the medial aspect of the sensory trigeminal root (V_3). The motor axons course deep to the trigeminal ganglion in the middle cranial fossa and leave the

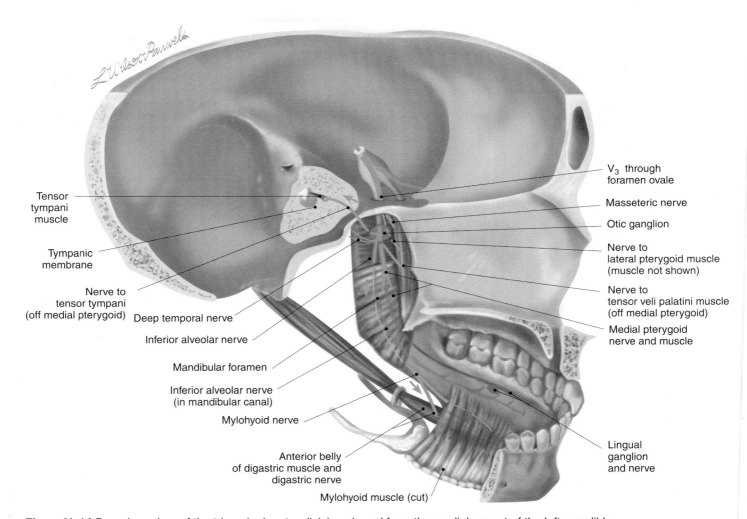

Figure V–14 Deep branches of the trigeminal motor division viewed from the medial aspect of the left mandible.

cranium through the foramen ovale (see Figure V–13). Just outside the foramen ovale they divide into five main branches: the medial and lateral pterygoid nerves, the masseteric nerve, the deep temporal nerves, and the mylohyoid nerve.

The *medial pterygoid nerve* gives off two small branches to the tensor veli palatini and tensor tympani and then enters the deep surface of the medial pterygoid muscle, which it supplies (see Figures V–13 and V–14).

The *lateral pterygoid nerve* runs briefly with the buccal nerve and enters the deep surface of the lateral pterygoid muscle.

The *masseteric nerve* passes laterally above the lateral pterygoid muscle through the mandibular notch to supply the masseter.

Two to three *deep temporal nerves* branch from the mandibular nerve, turn upwards, and pass superior to the lateral pterygoid muscle to enter the deep surface of the temporalis muscle.

The *mylohyoid nerve* travels with the inferior alveolar nerve, branching from it just before the latter enters the mandibular canal. The mylohyoid nerve continues anteriorly and inferiorly in a groove on the deep surface of the ramus of the mandible to reach the inferior surface of the mylohyoid muscle where it divides to supply the anterior belly of the digastric muscle and the mylohyoid muscle.

CASE HISTORY GUIDING QUESTIONS

1. What is trigeminal neuralgia?

2. What was Mary's family doctor looking for on the MRI scans?

3. Why are anticonvulsants effective in the treatment of trigeminal neuralgia?

4. Where along the trigeminal sensory and motor pathways can other pathologies occur?

5. What is the blink reflex, and why is it important?

1. What is trigeminal neuralgia?

Trigeminal neuralgia, also known as tic douloureux (painful spasm), is a condition in which excruciating paroxysms of pain occur in one or more divisions of the trigeminal nerve. The pain is typically lancinating in character and lasts a few seconds. The mandibular or maxillary divisions of the trigeminal nerve are most often involved, whereas the ophthalmic division is rarely involved. It is one of the most severe pains known in clinical medicine. The pain can occur spontaneously or can be elicited by eating, talking, shaving, brushing the teeth, or by touching a trigger zone. Trigeminal neuralgia patients often avoid these activities. To reduce sensory input from the mouth, many stop eating and may lose weight. They also protect their faces to avoid inadvertent touching. When the condition is severe, pain can occur many times an hour. Between attacks there is no pain, although patients live in dread of the next attack. Trigeminal neuralgia has an estimated incidence of 15 to 100 per 100,000 population. Women are twice as likely as men to develop this disease.

The precise mechanism of pain production is unknown but in some cases it is thought to be due to local irritation of the sensory fibers in the trigeminal nerve, which gives rise to spontaneous, ectopic impulses. A short high-frequency barrage of impulses is then projected to the cortex giving rise to the perception of severe pain.

2. What was Mary's family doctor looking for on the MRI scans?

Mary's doctor suspected that something was pressing on the root of her left trigeminal nerve causing the ectopic impulses that gave rise to her acutely painful sensations. The MRI scan showed a small meningioma in the middle cranial fossa adjacent to her trigeminal nerve root, which was the likely cause of her pain (Figure V–15). When tumors are present, trigeminal neuralgia may be associated with other neurologic findings because other anatomic structures in the brain stem are in close proximity and are easily compressed. In other cases, the trigeminal nerve can be irritated by the pulsations of a tortuous superior cerebellar artery.

3. Why are anticonvulsants effective in the treatment of trigeminal neuralgia?

Anticonvulsants act to decrease the firing rate of neurons. Carbamazepine is a sodium channel blocker that exerts its effect by decreasing the neuron's ability to

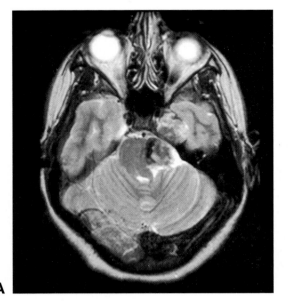
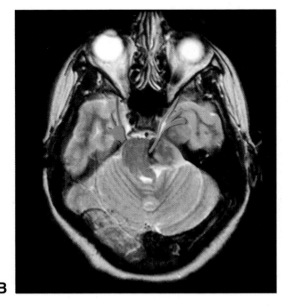

A   **B**

Figure V–15 Mary's MRI showed a meningioma growing on her left petrous temporal ridge. The tumor is pressing on her pons at the entry of the trigeminal nerve. *A*, MRI scan. *B*, The tumor has been artifically colored (*red*) and representations of the positions of the trigeminal nerves have been ghosted in to show that the left trigeminal nerve (*blue*) would be compressed by the meningioma. (Image courtesy of Dr. David Mikulis.)

produce a rapid train of impulses. Mary does not have epilepsy but, like epileptic patients, she does have an abnormal neuronal excitability. Mary's trigeminal neurons are hyperexcited because of the irritation caused by the meningeal tumor.

4. Where along the trigeminal sensory and motor pathways can other pathologies occur?

Pathology in the trigeminal system can occur anywhere along the course of the peripheral nerves, within the middle cranial fossa, or within the central nervous system.

Along the Course of the Peripheral Nerves

Branches of the trigeminal nerve can be damaged by injury to the head. The sensory and/or motor loss suffered depends on which branches are damaged. Herpes zoster (a virus infection commonly referred to as shingles) can invade the trigeminal ganglion where it can lie dormant. It can become active and travel along the peripheral processes, which leads to irritation during the outbreak and pain following resolution.

Within the Middle Cranial Fossa

As in Mary's case, the peripheral nerve can be damaged from compression by a meningioma as the nerve passes through the middle cranial fossa or by a schwannoma of the nerve itself. Schwannomas of the acoustic nerve, if sufficiently large, can also affect the trigeminal nerve causing pain and eventual loss of function. Because of their anatomic location at the junction of the cerebellum and the pons, acoustic neuromas give rise to a collection of symptoms (including trigeminal dysfunction) known as the cerebellopontine angle syndrome (Figure V–16) (see also Chapter VIII).

Within the Central Nervous System

Tumors and vascular problems can affect trigeminal pathways within the central nervous system (Figure V–17).

A. Within the medulla, damage to the trigeminal system gives rise primarily to loss of pain and temperature sensation on the ipsilateral (same) side of the face.

B. Within the pons, ipsilateral discriminative touch is primarily affected. Innervation of the ipsilateral muscles of mastication may also be affected, giving rise to a lower motor neuron lesion.

C. At levels of the neuraxis above the brain stem, all sensory modalities on the contralateral (opposite) side of the head are affected. Motor function is not affected because the motor (masticator) nucleus is driven by sensory reflex input from

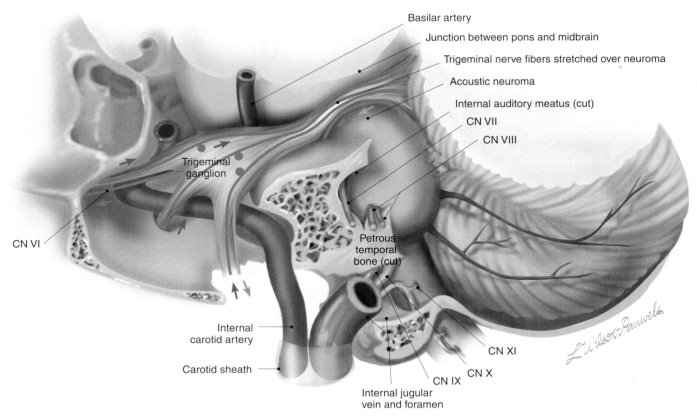

Basilar artery

Junction between pons and midbrain

Trigeminal nerve fibers stretched over neuroma

Acoustic neuroma

Internal auditory meatus (cut)

CN VII

CN VIII

Trigeminal ganglion

CN VI

Petrous temporal bone (cut)

Internal carotid artery

Carotid sheath

CN XI

CN X

CN IX

Internal jugular vein and foramen

Figure V–16 Acoustic neuroma: an enlarged tumor in the cerebellopontine angle compressing the root of the trigeminal nerve (sagittal section through the jugular foramen).

sensory neurons at the same level (see blink reflex, Figure V–18), and because it receives bilateral innervation from the cerebral hemispheres.

5. What is the blink reflex, and why is it important?

The blink reflex (see Figure V–18) is the closure of the eyes in response to certain stimuli (bright light, corneal irritation, and loud noise). The motor component of the blink reflex (closing the eyes) is mediated by the branchial motor fibers of the seventh cranial nerve (facial nerve). Several sensory pathways converge on the facial motor nucleus to activate the motor neurons. Initiating stimuli come from bright light via cranial nerve II, corneal stimulation via cranial nerve V (trigeminal), and loud sounds via cranial nerve VIII (auditory component).

Closing the eyes in response to intense light protects the retina from damage. Blinking in response to corneal irritation protects the cornea from airborne particles or other objects that could injure the eye. Blinking also prevents corneal dryness by moistening the cornea with tears. A dry cornea is painful and vulnerable to ulceration and infection. It is not certain why the eyes close in response to loud sounds, although presumably loud sounds could predict flying debris.

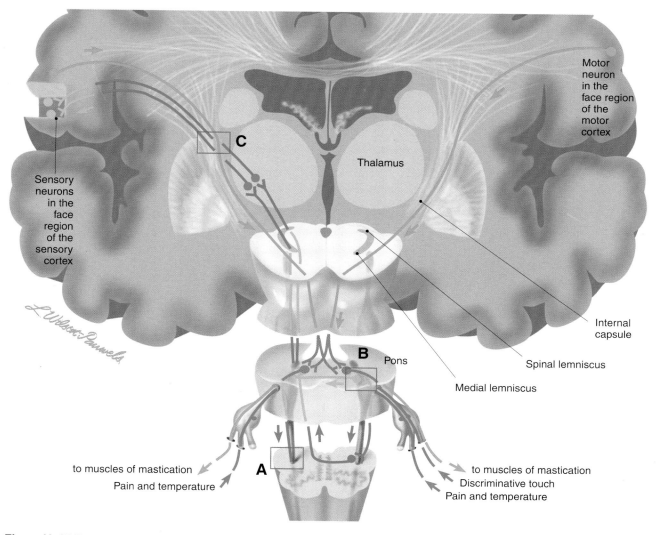

Figure V–17 Damage to the trigeminal pathways. *A*, Within the medulla; *B*, within the pons; and *C*, above the brain stem.

CLINICAL TESTING

When testing the trigeminal nerve, it is important to remember to test both the sensory and motor components. (See also Cranial Nerves Examination on CD-ROM.)

Sensory Component

The trigeminal nerve carries several sensory modalities, including discriminative touch, pain, temperature, and simple touch. All modalities are tested with the patient's eyes closed. When testing, the examiner first must check bilaterally for the presence of each modality in the forehead (V_1), cheeks (V_2), and jaw (V_3), and determine whether both sides of the face are equally sensitive (Figure V–19).

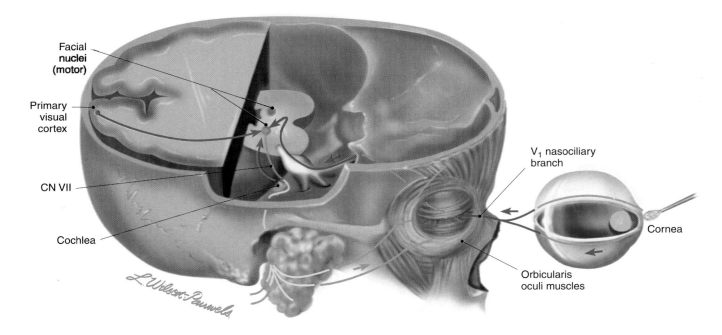

Figure V–18 Schematic rendering of the blink reflex (brain stem is elevated in response to touch).

The discriminative touch pathway is tested by touching the skin (gently) with the sharp end of a pointed object (ie, toothpick) and asking the patient what he or she feels. The pain and temperature pathway is tested by holding warm or cool objects against the skin. This can be done easily at the bedside by using the flat cool end of a tuning fork. Simple touch pathways are tested by lightly touching the skin with a wisp of cotton (see Figure V–19). The territories supplied by each division of the nerve are less variable in the central part of the face; therefore, testing should be done close to the midline.

The corneal reflex should always be tested when examining the trigeminal nerve. This test is particularly useful when assessing the integrity of V_1 in an unconscious patient. The corneal reflex is tested by observing whether the patient blinks in response to a light touch with a wisp of cotton on the cornea, not the sclera (see Figure V–18).

Motor Component

To test the motor component of the trigeminal nerve, the examiner palpates the masseter and temporalis muscles on both sides and asks the patient to clamp the jaws tightly together. The examiner should feel the contraction of each muscle. The patient is then asked to open his or her mouth so that the examiner can look for jaw deviation. If the motor component is not functioning correctly, the jaw will deviate toward the weak side. The patient is then asked to move the jaw to one side while the examiner attempts to push it back to the midline position. The examiner should

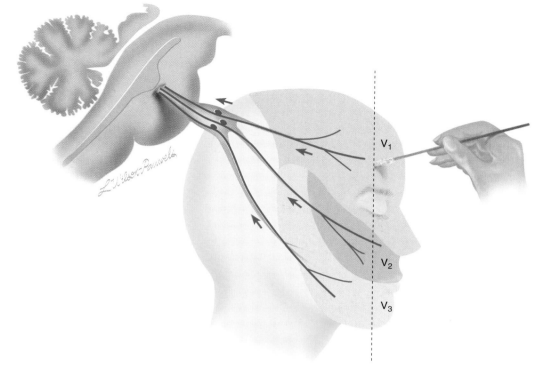

Figure V–19 Clinical testing for sensation.

not be able to overcome the strength of the pterygoid muscles. This is repeated on the other side.

To complete the motor examination, the jaw jerk should be tested. The mandibular (jaw jerk) reflex can be tested by tapping the middle of the chin with a reflex hammer while the patient's mouth is slightly open. A sudden slight closing of the jaw constitutes a normal reflex.

ADDITIONAL RESOURCES

Collins RC. Neurology. Toronto: W.B. Saunders Co.; 1997. p. 43.

DeJong RN, Sahs AL, Aldrich CK, Milligan JO. Essentials of the neurological examination. Philadelphia: Smith Kline Corporation; 1979.

Fromm GH. The pharmacology of trigeminal neuralgia. Clin Neuropharmacol 1989;12: 185–94.

Fromm GH. Trigeminal neuralgia and related disorders. Neurol Clin 1989;7:305–19.

Fromm GH. Clinical pharmacology of drugs used to treat head and face pain. Neurol Clin 1990;8:143–51.

Hamlyn PJ, King TT. Neurovascular compression in trigeminal neuralgia: a clinical and anatomical study. J Neurosurg 1992;76:948–54.

Harsh GR, Wilson CB, Hieshima GB, Dillon WP. Magnetic resonance imaging of verte-brobasilar ectasia in tic convulsif. Case report. J Neurosurg 1991;74:999–1003.

Kandel RR, Schwartz JH, Jessell TM. Principles of neural science. 3rd ed. New York: Elsevier; 1991. p. 703–5.

Lindsay KW, Bone I, Callander R. Neurology and neurosurgery illustrated. 2nd ed. New York: Churchill Livingstone; 1991. p. 159.

Macdonald RL, Meldrum BS. Principles of antiepileptic drug action. In: Levy R, Mattson R, Meldrum B, et al, editors. Antiepileptic drugs. New York: Raven Press Ltd.; 1989. p. 59–83.

Sidebottom A, Maxwell S. The medical and surgical management of trigeminal neuralgia. J Clin Pharm Ther 1995;20:31–5.

Taurig HH, Maley BE. The trigeminal system. In: Conn PM, editor. Neuroscience in medicine. Philadelphia: JB Lippincott; 1995. p. 239–48.

Walton J. Introduction to clinical neuroscience. 2nd ed. Toronto: Baillière Tindall; 1987. p. 209–10.

VI Abducens Nerve

*innervates
the
lateral rectus
muscle
of the eye*

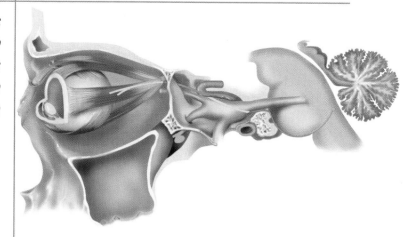

VI Abducens Nerve

CASE HISTORY

Grace is a 36-year-old editor of a Hong Kong–based travel magazine. Grace had been well until about three months ago when she began having intermittent nosebleeds. The first nosebleed bled heavily for about 1 hour and stopped on its own. Since this first incident, Grace has had two further nosebleeds. About 2 months ago she noticed that she had double vision when she looked to the left. Initially it was intermittent, but it soon became a persistent problem. In the last month, she developed numbness of her left upper lip that spread to her left cheek and then to her forehead. Grace had been trying to ignore these symptoms, but when she had another bad nosebleed, she went to the emergency department of a nearby hospital.

Within 15 minutes of her arrival in the emergency department, Grace's nosebleed had stopped. She explained her recent symptoms to the doctor, who then called a neurologist. When the neurologist examined Grace, he found that her pupils were equal and reactive to light, and that there was no evidence of ptosis (upper eyelid droop). The movements of her right eye were normal, but Grace clearly had problems moving her left eye. It was found that Grace was unable to abduct her left eye (look to the left) and when she attempted to do so, would see a double image. However, she could look in all other directions without difficulty. When the neurologist tested for sensation on Grace's face, he found that she had numbness on her left forehead, cheek, and upper lip, while her lower lip and chin had normal sensation. Grace had symmetric facial movements and there was no evidence of weakness of her facial muscles. The remainder of her cranial nerves were functioning normally.

The doctor was concerned that Grace had a lesion involving her cavernous sinus, so he ordered a computed tomography (CT) scan of her head. The scan demonstrated a mass from the pharynx infiltrating upwards into the cavernous sinus. The doctor suspected that Grace might have a nasopharyngeal carcinoma and, therefore, arranged for an otolaryngologist to obtain a biopsy of the suspicious mass.

ANATOMY OF THE ABDUCENS NERVE

The abducens nerve has only a somatic motor component (Figure VI–1). The function of this cranial nerve is to move the eye laterally away from the midline (Table VI–1) (the name is from the Latin words *ab* [away] and *ducere* [to lead]). Axons of the abducens nerve emerge from the ventral aspect of the brain stem at the pontomedullary junction. The nerve runs rostrally and slightly laterally in the subarachnoid space of the posterior cranial fossa to pierce the dura at a point lateral to the dorsum sellae of the sphenoid bone (Figure VI–2). It continues forward between the dura and the apex of the petrous temporal bone where it takes a sharp right-angled bend over the apex and enters the cavernous sinus. Within the cavernous

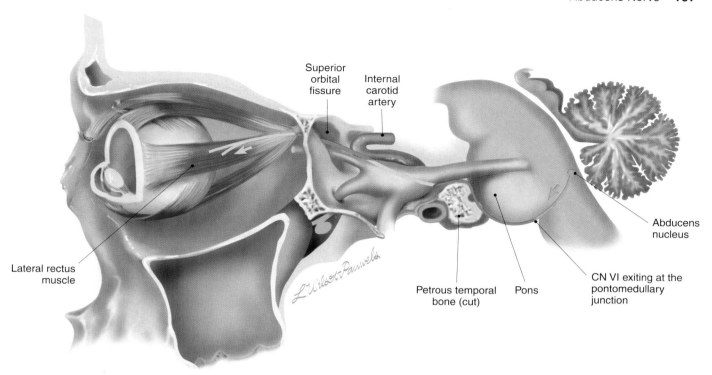

Figure VI–1 Overview of the abducens nerve.

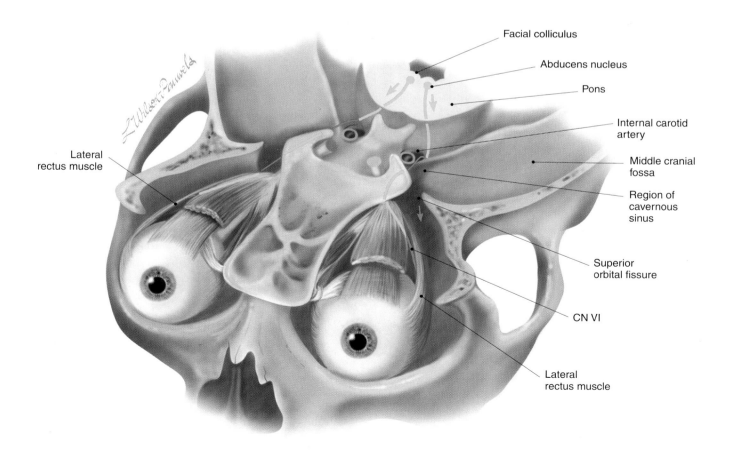

Figure VI–2 Route of the abducens nerve (cranial nerve VI) from the pons to the lateral rectus muscle.

Table VI–1 Nerve Fiber Modality and Function of the Abducens Nerve

Nerve Fiber Modality	Nucleus	Function
Somatic motor (efferent)	Abducens	Innervation of the lateral rectus muscle of the eye

sinus, the sixth nerve is situated lateral to the internal carotid artery and medial to cranial nerves III, IV, V_1, and V_2 (Figure VI–3). Continuing forward, the abducens nerve leaves the cavernous sinus and enters the orbit at the medial end of the superior orbital fissure. It is then encircled by the tendinous ring, which provides a point of origin for the four recti muscles of the eye. The nerve enters the deep surface of the lateral rectus muscle, which it supplies (Table VI–2 and Figure VI–4).

The Abducens Nucleus

The abducens nucleus is located in the pons. Like other somatic motor nuclei, the abducens nucleus is situated close to the midline. The nucleus is composed of two kinds of cells: lower motor neurons, whose axons constitute the abducens nerve, and internuclear neurons, which project via the medial longitudinal fasciculus (MLF) to medial rectus lower motor neurons in the contralateral oculomotor nucleus. These are important for coordination of the lateral gaze (see Chapter 13). Axons of the lower motor neurons in the abducens nucleus course ventrally through the pons to emerge from the ventral surface of the brain stem at the pontomedullary junction (see Figure VI–1 and Figure VI–5).

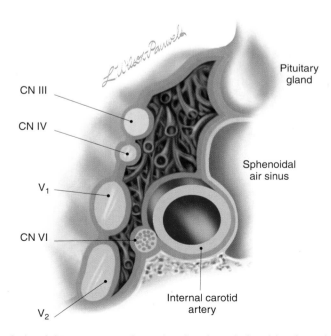

Figure VI–3 Slice through the right cavernous sinus showing the relationship of cranial nerve VI to other structures coursing through the sinus.

Table VI–2 Eye Movements Mediated by Cranial Nerve VI

Nerve	Muscle	Primary Action	Subsidiary Action
CN VI	Lateral rectus	Abduction	None

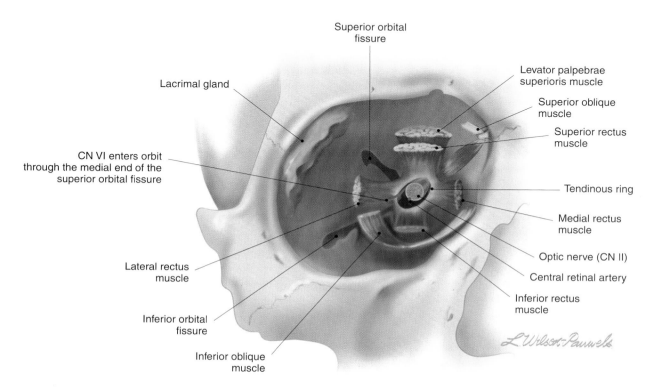

Figure VI–4 Apex of the right orbit illustrating the tendinous ring and the somatic motor component of cranial nerve VI.

CASE HISTORY GUIDING QUESTIONS

1. Why was Grace having nosebleeds?

2. Why did Grace have double vision only when she was looking to the left?

3. How did the doctor know that the problem was within the cavernous sinus?

4. Why did Grace not have a numb chin?

5. Where else along the course of cranial nerve VI could damage occur?

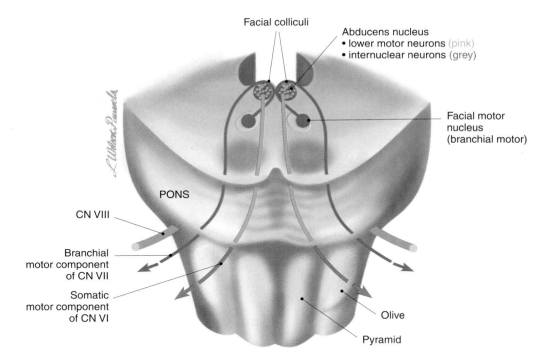

Facial colliculi

Abducens nucleus
• lower motor neurons (pink)
• internuclear neurons (grey)

Facial motor
nucleus
(branchial motor)

PONS

CN VIII

Branchial
motor component
of CN VII

Somatic
motor component
of CN VI

Olive

Pyramid

Figure VI–5 Abducens nuclei in the brain stem. Branchial motor axons from the facial nucleus loop over the abducens nucleus thereby creating an elevation (bump) in the floor of the fourth ventricle, called the facial colliculus. Because of this close anatomic association, lesions of the facial colliculus affect both cranial nerve VI and cranial nerve VII.

1. Why was Grace having nosebleeds?

The veins of the nose, including those of the highly vascular nasal mucosa, drain posteriorly into the cavernous sinus. The mass in Grace's posterior pharynx was invading her cavernous sinus, interfering with blood flow, and causing venous congestion in her nasal mucosa. The increased blood pressure within the delicate mucous membranes caused the small blood vessels to rupture and thus caused her nose to bleed.

2. Why did Grace have double vision only when she was looking to the left?

Horizontal eye movements require the coordinated action of the medial and lateral rectus muscles. The doctor noticed that when Grace attempted to look to the left, her left eye was unable to abduct (Figure VI–6). This led him to conclude that Grace's left lateral rectus muscle was weak. On attempting leftward gaze, Grace was unable to align both eyes toward the same target. Therefore, the visual fields were projected onto different areas of the right and left retinae, and two images were seen. Looking to the right and in the midline does not require the action of the left lateral rectus muscle; therefore, Grace's vision was normal in these directions.

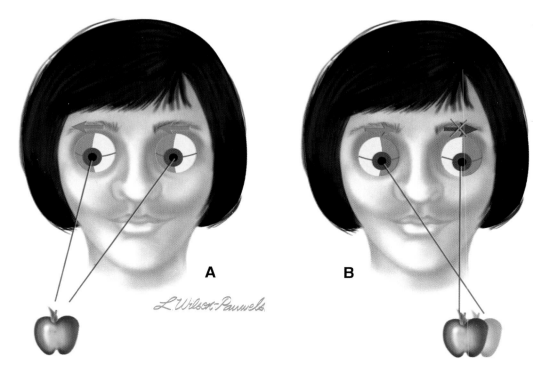

Figure VI–6 *A*, When looking to the right, Grace was able to direct both eyes toward the same object. *B*, On attempted left lateral gaze, Grace was unable to abduct her left eye due to paralysis of her left lateral rectus muscle; therefore, she experienced double vision.

3. How did the doctor know that the problem was within the cavernous sinus?

The first step to solving this problem is to identify the nerves involved. Grace was unable to abduct her left eye. The lateral rectus muscle, which is responsible for eye abduction, is innervated by cranial nerve VI. Therefore, either her left lateral rectus muscle or her left cranial nerve VI is involved. Grace also had numbness over her left forehead and cheek. The ophthalmic division of the trigeminal nerve (V_1) supplies sensation to the forehead, the maxillary division of the trigeminal nerve (V_2) supplies sensation to the cheek, and the mandibular division of the trigeminal nerve (V_3) supplies sensation to the chin (see Chapter V). Therefore, the left V_1 and V_2 are also affected but the left V_3 is spared.

The second step to solving the problem involves a knowledge of the anatomy of the cranial nerves. It is reasonable to assume there is only one cause for Grace's problem and, therefore, that the site of the lesion is located where cranial nerve VI and cranial nerves V_1 and V_2 are in close proximity to each other. The only anatomic place where this occurs is within the cavernous sinus (see Figure VI–3). Therefore, disease processes of the cavernous sinus can affect these nerves.

4. Why did Grace not have a numb chin?

The mandibular division of the trigeminal nerve (V_3) passes just outside the cavernous sinus and, therefore, was not involved by the infiltrating mass.

5. Where else along the course of cranial nerve VI could damage occur?

Cranial nerve VI can be damaged anywhere along its course from its nucleus in the pons to its target muscle in the orbit (the lateral rectus muscle).

Within the Brain Stem

The nucleus and its axons can be affected by infarction, tumor, or demyelination.

Once it has Left the Brain Stem

The nerve itself can become ischemic (this is most commonly seen in patients with diabetes or hypertension). The nerve can be affected by meningeal infection. Occasionally cerebellopontine angle tumors can involve cranial nerve VI as well as cranial nerves V, VII, and VIII (see Chapter VIII, Figure VIII–3). Mastoiditis (inflammation of the mastoid process of the temporal bone) can involve cranial nerve V as well as cranial nerve VI (Gradenigo's syndrome).

Within the Cavernous Sinus

As cranial nerve VI passes anteriorly through the cavernous sinus, the nerve can be involved in any disease process within the sinus (carotid aneurysm, sinus thrombosis, infection, inflammation, or tumor). Other cranial nerves are commonly affected at this site (III, IV, V_1, V_2) due to their close proximity within the cavernous sinus.

Within the Superior Orbital Fissure

Cranial nerve VI passes anteriorly through the superior orbital fissure to reach the lateral rectus muscle. Fractures of the orbit or orbital tumors could compromise the nerve. Other cranial nerves (III, IV, and V_1) passing through the fissure also can be affected.

CLINICAL TESTING

Cranial nerve VI is tested in conjunction with cranial nerves III and IV through the assessment of eye movements (See Chapter 13). When testing specifically for cranial nerve VI, it is important to bring the eye through the full extent of the horizontal plane and to ensure that the eye moves fully away from the midline (Figure VI–7). (See also Cranial Nerves Examination on CD-ROM.)

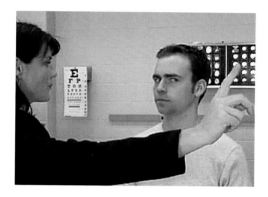

Figure VI–7 Testing the abducens nerve.

ADDITIONAL RESOURCES

Brodal A. Neurological anatomy in relation to clinical medicine. 3rd ed. New York: Oxford University Press; 1981. p. 532–77.

Büttner U, Büttner-Ennever JA. Present concepts of oculomotor organization. In: Büttner-Ennever JA, editor. Neuroanatomy of the oculomotor system. Amsterdam: Elsevier; 1988. p. 3–32.

Glimcher PA. Eye movements. In: Zigmond MJ, Bloom FE, Landis SC, et al, editors. Fundamental neuroscience. San Diego: Academic Press; 1999. p. 993–1009.

Goldberg MW. The control of gaze. In: Kandel ER, Schwartz JH, Jessell TM, editors. Principles of neural science. 4th ed. New York: McGraw Hill; 2000. p. 782–800.

Goldberg ME, Hudspeth AJ. The vestibular system. In: Kandel ER, Schwartz JH, Jessell TM, editors. Principles of neural science. 4th ed. New York: McGraw Hill; 2000. p. 801–15.

Leigh RJ, Zee DS. The neurology of eye movements. 3rd ed. New York: Oxford University Press; 1999. p. 3–15.

VII Facial Nerve

carries general sensation from the ear, carries the special sense of taste, and innervates the muscles of facial expression and the sublingual, submandibular, and lacrimal glands

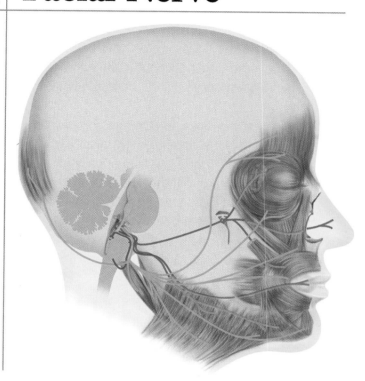

VII Facial Nerve

CASE HISTORY

John is a 45-year-old man in the prime of his career. One morning he was having some difficulties shaving that resulted in a couple of nicks on the right side of his face. He went to work and, at lunch time, ordered soup because his mouth felt unusually dry. To his embarrassment, the soup dribbled out of the right corner of his mouth. After lunch, he looked in the mirror and noticed that the entire right side of his face was drooping, but otherwise his face felt normal. John phoned his family doctor who arranged to see him that afternoon.

At the end of the day when the family doctor saw John, he was unable to raise his right eyebrow or completely close his right eye. Neither was he able to raise the right corner of his mouth, and, as a result, his face appeared to be pulled to the left. The doctor also discovered that John had lost the ability to taste anything on the anterior two-thirds of his tongue on the right side. There was no change in sensation on his face and his hearing was normal, but there was a lot of tearing of the right eye. The rest of John's cranial nerves were functioning normally. John's doctor diagnosed Bell's palsy, assured him that he should make a good recovery, and started him on an appropriate medication.

Despite expectations, six weeks later there was no apparent change, but by eight months after the onset, the right side of John's face was almost back to normal. John saw his doctor again who observed an interesting phenomenon. Every time John smiled, his right eye would close. There were no other apparent abnormalities and John was reassured by his doctor that this unusual motor activity was a consequence of the Bell's palsy, and that he was otherwise normal.

ANATOMY OF THE FACIAL NERVE

The facial nerve is the most frequently paralyzed of all the peripheral nerves. Figure VII–1 provides a diagrammatic overview of the facial nerve components and their locations. As well, an overview of their functional relationships is provided in Table VII–1. The branchial motor fibers (sometimes called the facial nerve proper) are adjacent to (medial), but separated from, the remaining fibers. The remaining fibers carrying visceral motor and general and special sensory information, are bound in a distinct fascial sheath and are referred to as *nervus intermedius* (Figure VII–2).

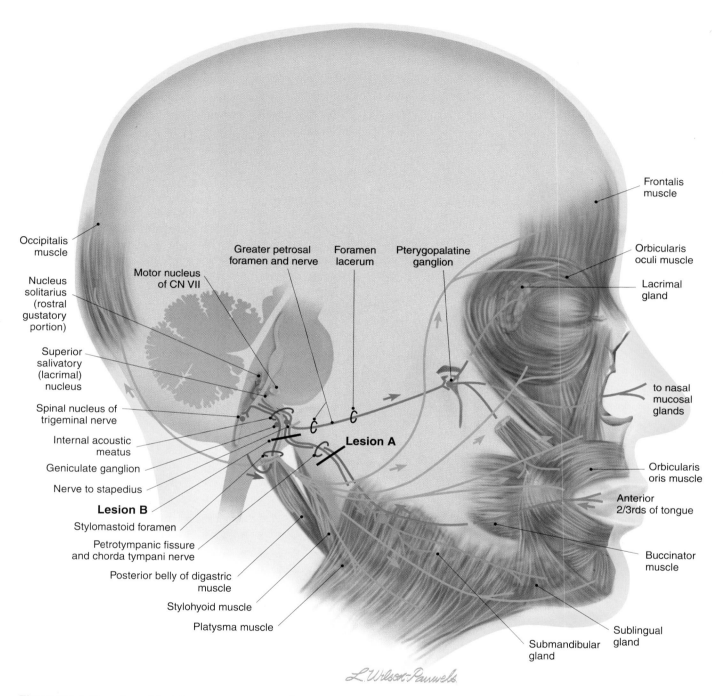

Occipitalis
muscle

Nucleus
solitarius
(rostral
gustatory
portion)

Superior
salivatory
(lacrimal)
nucleus

Spinal nucleus of
trigeminal nerve

Internal acoustic
meatus

Geniculate ganglion

Nerve to stapedius

Lesion B

Stylomastoid foramen

Petrotympanic fissure
and chorda tympani nerve

Posterior belly of digastric
muscle

Stylohyoid muscle

Platysma muscle

Motor nucleus
of CN VII

Greater petrosal
foramen and nerve

Foramen
lacerum

Pterygopalatine
ganglion

Lesion A

Frontalis
muscle

Orbicularis
oculi muscle

Lacrimal
gland

to nasal
mucosal
glands

Orbicularis
oris muscle

Anterior
2/3rds of tongue

Buccinator
muscle

Sublingual
gland

Submandibular
gland

L. Wilson-Pauwels

Figure VII–1 Overview of facial nerve components (parotid gland removed).

Table VII–1 Nerve Fiber Modality and Function of the Facial Nerve

Nerve Fiber Modality	Nucleus	Function
General sensory (afferent)	Spinal of the trigeminal nerve	To carry sensation from the skin of the concha of the auricle, a small area of skin behind the ear, and possibly to supplement V_3, which carries sensation from the wall of the external auditory meatus and the external surface of the tympanic membrane
Special sensory (afferent)	Solitarius (rostral gustatory portion)	For taste sensation from the anterior two-thirds of the tongue
Branchial motor (efferent)	Motor of cranial nerve VII	To supply the muscles of facial expression (ie, frontalis, occipitalis, orbicularis oculi, corrugator supercilii, procerus, nasalis, levator labii superiorus, levator labii superioris alaeque nasi, zygomaticus major and minor, levator anguli oris, mentalis, depressor labii inferioris, depressor anguli oris, buccinator, orbicularis oris, risorius, and platysma). In addition, the branchial motor fibers supply the stapedius, stylohyoid, and posterior belly of digastric muscles
Visceral motor (parasympathetic efferent)	Superior salivatory (lacrimal)	For stimulation of the lacrimal, submandibular, and sublingual glands as well as the mucous membrane of the nose and hard and soft palates

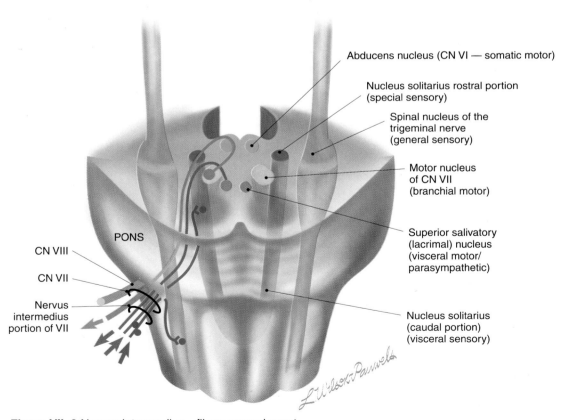

Figure VII–2 Nervus intermedius—fibers spread apart.

Course of the Facial Nerve

Cranial nerve VII emerges from the brain stem at the lower border of the pons, crosses the subarachnoid space, and enters the internal acoustic meatus (Figures VII–1 and VII–3). In its course through the petrous part of the temporal bone, the facial nerve displays a swelling, the *geniculate ganglion*, containing the nerve cell bodies of the taste axons from the tongue and of the somatic sensory axons from the external ear, auditory meatus, and external surface of the tympanic membrane. At the geniculate ganglion, the facial nerve gives off the parasympathetic greater petrosal nerve that courses anteriorly to the pterygopalatine ganglion. The remaining axons then continue along the facial canal where the chorda tympani nerve branches off. It carries taste sensations in from, and parasympathetic motor fibers out to, the tongue and oral cavity. The general sensory and branchial motor fibers of the facial nerve finally emerge from the skull through the stylomastoid foramen and pass forward through the substance of the parotid gland to supply the muscles of facial expression.

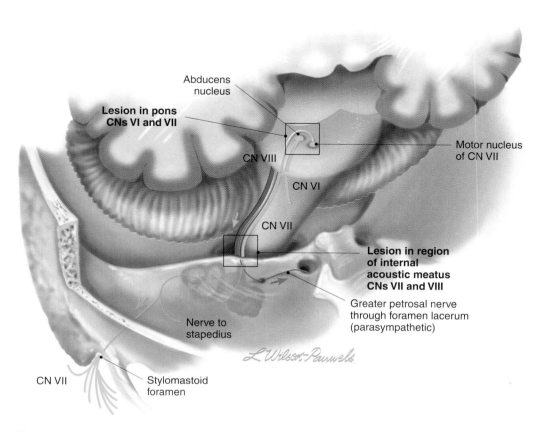

Figure VII–3 Lesion in pons versus lesion in internal acoustic meatus—brain stem is elevated.

GENERAL SENSORY (AFFERENT) COMPONENT

Cranial nerve VII has a small cutaneous sensory component that is found in the nervus intermedius (Figure VII–4). Cutaneous nerve endings can be found around the skin of the concha and the posteromedial surface of the pinna of the external ear and in a small area behind the ear. This nerve possibly supplements the mandibular nerve (V_3) by providing sensation from the wall of the external acoustic meatus and the external surface of the tympanic membrane.

These afferent fibers join the branchial motor axons of the facial nerve at the sylomastoid foramen and travel centrally. Their nerve cell bodies are located in the *geniculate ganglion* in the petrous part of the temporal bone. Impulses from this ganglion enter the brain stem via the nervus intermedius to reach the *spinal tract of the trigeminal nerve* where they descend to synapse in the spinal portion of the trigem-

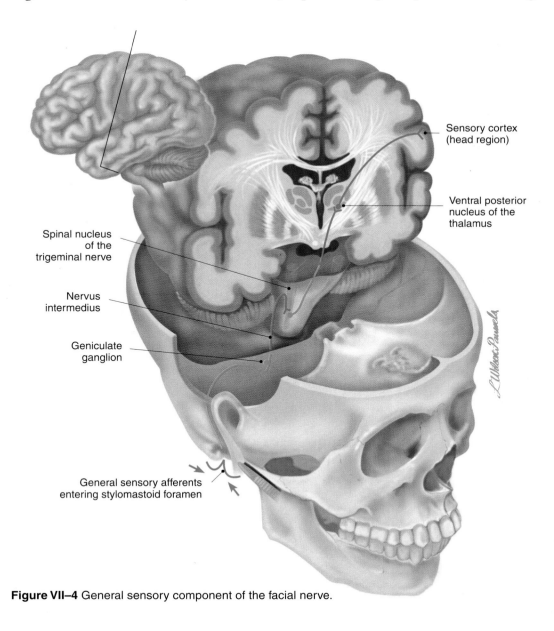

Figure VII–4 General sensory component of the facial nerve.

inal nucleus in the upper medulla. From this nucleus, impulses are projected to the contralateral ventral posterior nucleus of the thalamus; from there, tertiary sensory neurons project to the sensory cortex of the postcentral gyrus (head region).

SPECIAL SENSORY (AFFERENT) COMPONENT

Special sensory fibers of cranial nerve VII carry information from the taste buds on the lateral border of the anterior two-thirds of the tongue and the hard and soft palates (Figure VII–5). Peripheral processes of these cells for taste run with the lingual nerve and separate from it to join the chorda tympani.

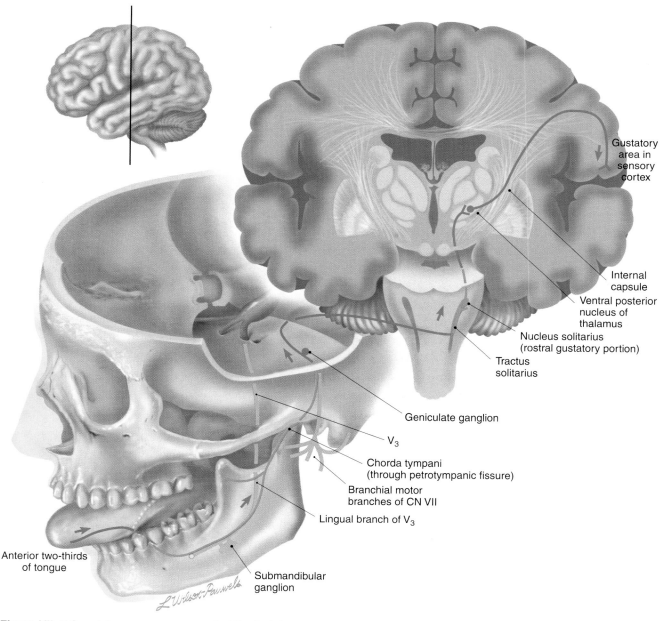

Figure VII–5 Special sensory component of the facial nerve.

The chorda tympani enters the petrotympanic fissure and joins the facial nerve in the petrous part of the temporal bone. The cell bodies of the special sensory neurons for taste are located in the geniculate ganglion on the medial wall of the tympanic cavity. From the ganglion, fibers enter the brain stem at the caudal border of the pons with the other fibers of the nervus intermedius. They then enter the *tractus solitarius* in the brain stem and synapse in the rostral portion of the *nucleus solitarius*, which is sometimes identified as the *gustatory nucleus*.

Unlike other sensory projections, the ascending (secondary) fibers from this nucleus project ipsilaterally via the central tegmental tract to reach the ipsilateral ventral posterior nucleus of the thalamus. Axons of thalamic (tertiary) neurons then project through the posterior limb of the internal capsule to the cortical area for taste, which is located in the most inferior part of the sensory cortex in the postcentral gyrus and extends onto the insula.

BRANCHIAL MOTOR (EFFERENT) COMPONENT

Signals for voluntary movements of the facial muscles originate in the cerebral cortex. They travel through the posterior limb of the internal capsule as part of the corticobulbar tract and project to the ispilateral and contralateral motor nuclei of cranial nerve VII in the tegmentum of the caudal pons. The branchial motor component is illustrated in Figure VII–6.

Upper motor neurons that project to the part of the nucleus innervating the forehead muscles project bilaterally, but those that project to the part of the nucleus innervating the remaining facial muscles project only contralaterally (Figures VII–7 and VII–8).

The branchial motor axons of the facial nerve form the efferent component of several reflex arcs. These are closing the eye in response to touching the cornea (corneal reflex) or to bright light (light reflex); contraction or relaxation of the stapedius muscles in response to sound intensity (stapedius reflex); and sucking-in response to touch sensations in the mouth (sucking reflex). As well, the facial muscles respond to emotional input as seen in the characteristic facial expressions in response to strong emotions such as rage or joy. The pathways for emotionally driven facial expressions are not yet known but probably include the limbic system and basal ganglia connections within the forebrain. Patients with Parkinson's disease have the same difficulty driving facial movements as they do with other types of motor activity. As a result, they have a characteristic, apparently emotionless, expression.

After synapsing in the motor nucleus, the axons of the lower motor neurons course dorsally toward the floor of the fourth ventricle and loop around the abducens nucleus to form a slight bulge in the floor of the fourth ventricle—the *facial colliculus* (see FigureVII–7). The loop itself is the *internal genu* of the facial nerve. These fibers then turn ventrally to emerge on the ventrolateral aspect of the brain stem at the caudal border of the pons, between the sixth and eighth cranial nerves and medial to the nervus intermedius portion of the seventh cranial nerve (see Figure VII–2).

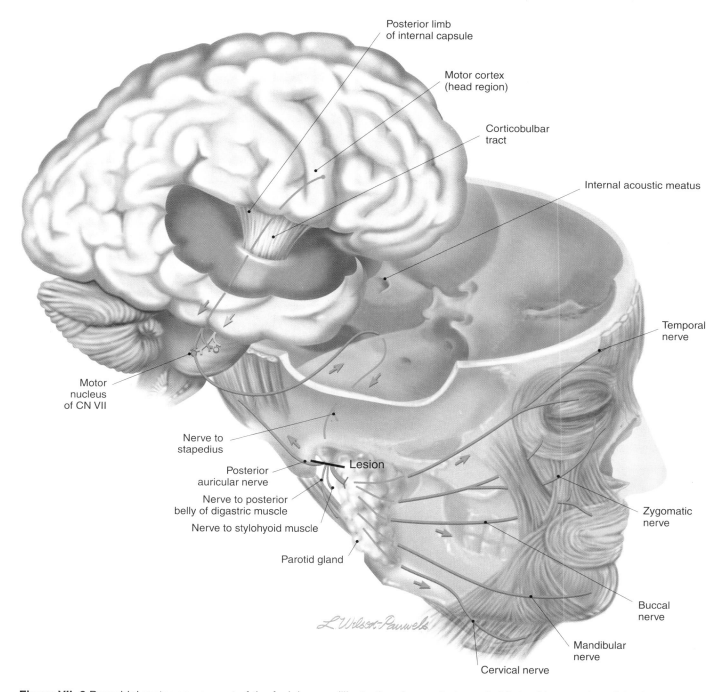

Posterior limb
of internal capsule

Motor cortex
(head region)

Corticobulbar
tract

Internal acoustic meatus

Temporal
nerve

Motor
nucleus
of CN VII

Nerve to
stapedius

Lesion

Posterior
auricular nerve

Nerve to posterior
belly of digastric muscle

Nerve to stylohyoid muscle

Parotid gland

Zygomatic
nerve

Buccal
nerve

Mandibular
nerve

Cervical nerve

Figure VII–6 Branchial motor component of the facial nerve (illustration demonstrates only bilateral innervation of the facial nucleus).

Branchial motor axons from neurons of cranial nerve VII accompany cranial nerve VIII through the internal auditory meatus to enter the petrous part of the temporal bone. The fibers lie within the facial canal of the temporal bone between the organs of hearing and equilibrium and then turn laterally and caudally in the facial canal (see Figure VII–3). The *nerve to stapedius* is given off here. Branchial motor fibers exit the

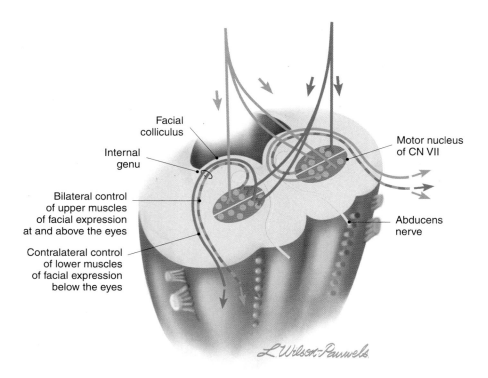

Figure VII–7 Motor nucleus of cranial nerve VII in the pons.

facial canal at the stylomastoid foramen and immediately give branches to the stylo-hyoid and the posterior belly of digastric muscles, and form the posterior auricular nerve to the occipitalis muscle. The remaining branchial motor fibers pass anteriorly to pierce and lie within the substance of the parotid gland. At this point the nerve divides into the temporal, zygomatic, buccal, mandibular, and cervical branches to supply the muscles of the scalp, face, and neck (see Figure VII–6 and Table VII–2).

Table VII–2 Facial Nerve Branches to Face and Neck Muscles

Named Branches	Muscles Supplied
Nerve to stapedius	Stapedius
Nerve to posterior belly of digastric	Posterior belly of digastric
Nerve to stylohyoid	Stylohyoid
Temporal	Frontalis, occipitalis, orbicularis oculi, corrugator supercilii, procerus
Zygomatic	Orbicularis oculi
Buccal	Buccinator, orbicularis oris, nasalis, levator labii superioris, levator labii superioris alaeque nasi, zygomaticus major and minor, levator anguli oris
Mandibular	Orbicularis oris, mentalis, depressor anguli oris, depressor labii inferioris, risorius
Cervical	Platysma
Posterior auricular	Occipitalis

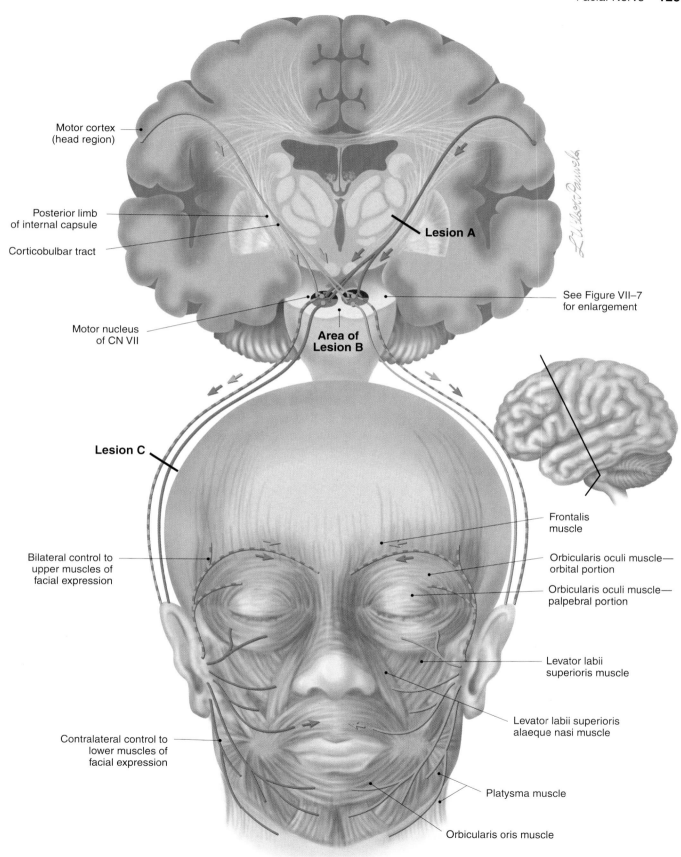

Motor cortex (head region)

Posterior limb of internal capsule

Corticobulbar tract

Lesion A

See Figure VII–7 for enlargement

Motor nucleus of CN VII

Area of Lesion B

Lesion C

Frontalis muscle

Orbicularis oculi muscle— orbital portion

Orbicularis oculi muscle— palpebral portion

Bilateral control to upper muscles of facial expression

Levator labii superioris muscle

Levator labii superioris alaeque nasi muscle

Contralateral control to lower muscles of facial expression

Platysma muscle

Orbicularis oris muscle

Figure VII–8 Bilateral (dotted lines) and contralateral (solid lines) projections from the facial nuclei.

VISCERAL MOTOR
(PARASYMPATHETIC EFFERENT) COMPONENT

An important part of cranial nerve VII is its *parasympathetic* component that is responsible for control of the lacrimal, submandibular, and sublingual glands and mucous glands of the nose, paranasal sinuses, and hard and soft palates (ie, all the major glands of the head except the integumentary glands and the parotid gland). The cell bodies (preganglionic autonomic motor neurons) are scattered in the pontine tegmentum and are collectively called the *superior salivatory nucleus* (sometimes known as the lacrimal nucleus). The visceral motor component is illustrated in Figure VII–9.

The superior salivatory nucleus is influenced primarily by the hypothalamus, an important controlling and integrating center of the autonomic nervous system. Impulses from the limbic system (emotional behavior) and the olfactory area (special

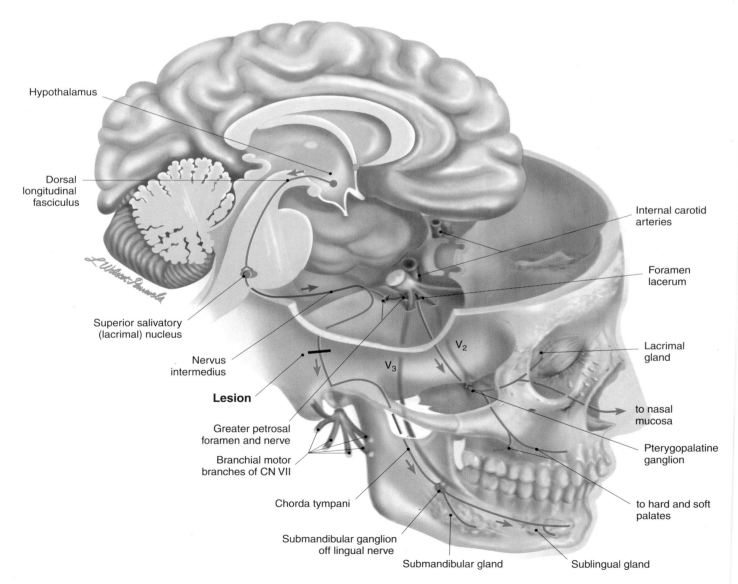

Figure VII–9 Visceral motor component of the facial nerve.

sensory area for smell) enter the hypothalamus and are relayed via the *dorsal longitudinal fasciculus* to the *superior salivatory (lacrimal) nucleus*. These pathways mediate visceral reflexes such as salivation in response to odors (eg, to cooking odors) or weeping in response to emotional states.

The superior salivatory nucleus is also influenced by other areas of the brain. For example, when the eye is irritated, sensory fibers travel to the spinal trigeminal nucleus in the brain stem, which, in turn, stimulates the superior salivatory nucleus to cause secretion of the lacrimal gland (see Figure VII–9). When special taste fibers in the mouth are activated, the nucleus solitarius (rostral gustatory portion) stimulates the superior salivatory nucleus to cause secretion of the oral glands.

The efferent fibers from the superior salivatory nucleus travel in the *nervus intermedius*. They divide at the geniculate ganglion in the facial canal into two groups to become the *greater petrosal nerve* (to the lacrimal and nasal glands) and part of the *chorda tympani nerve* (to submandibular and sublingual glands).

The *greater petrosal nerve* exits the petrous portion of the temporal bone via the greater petrosal foramen to enter the middle cranial fossa. It passes deep to the trigeminal ganglion to reach the foramen lacerum. It helps to think of the foramen lacerum as a short vertical chimney. The greater petrosal nerve traverses the lateral wall of the chimney to reach the pterygoid canal. Here it joins with the deep petrosal nerve (sympathetic fibers from the plexus that surrounds the internal carotid artery) to become the *nerve of the pterygoid canal* (Figure VII–10). This canal is

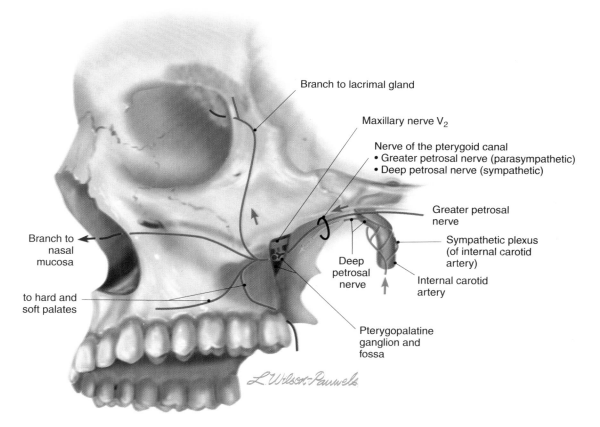

Figure VII–10 Nerve of the pterygoid canal.

located in the base of the medial pterygoid plate of the sphenoid bone and opens into the pterygopalatine fossa where the *pterygopalatine ganglion* is located. Axons of parasympathetic neurons in the nerve of the pterygoid canal synapse in the parasympathetic pterygopalatine ganglion. Postganglionic fibers continue forward, some with branches of V_2, to reach the lacrimal gland and the mucous glands in the mucosa of the nasal and oral cavities where they stimulate secretion.

The *chorda tympani nerve* passes through the petrotympanic fissure to join the lingual branch of the mandibular nerve (V_3) after the latter has passed through the foramen ovale. These two nerve bundles travel together toward the lateral border of the floor of the oral cavity where the parasympathetic fibers of cranial nerve VII synapse in the submandibular ganglion that is suspended from the lingual nerve. Postganglionic fibers continue to the submandibular and sublingual glands and to minor glands in the floor of the mouth where they stimulate secretion.

CASE HISTORY GUIDING QUESTIONS

1. What is Bell's palsy and what causes this disorder?

2. Why did John have trouble contracting the muscles on the right side of his face and neck?

3. Why was John's mouth dry?

4. What is the anatomic basis for the loss of taste to the anterior two-thirds of John's tongue on the right side?

5. How do substances in John's mouth give rise to electrical signals in gustatory neurons?

6. What is the anatomic basis of John's excessive tearing?

7. How does an understanding of John's excessive tearing problem help you to locate the site of the lesion?

8. Why was John's recovery so prolonged?

9. Why does John's right eye close every time he smiles?

10. What other lesions could affect the motor component of the facial nerve?

1. What is Bell's palsy and what causes this disorder?

Bell's palsy is paralysis of the facial nerve of unknown cause (idiopathic). It occurs most frequently in the facial canal of the petrous portion of the temporal bone. It affects both men and women equally and the incidence is 23 per 100,000 annually. The signs and symptoms of Bell's palsy are determined by which branches of the facial nerve are affected. Facial nerve palsy can involve the motor, secretory, and sensory components. The primary symptom in involvement of the motor branch is acute onset of unilateral weakness reaching its maximum paralysis in 48 to 72 hours. Impairment of taste and hyperacusis (sounds seem louder than normal) can occur from involvement of the chorda tympani nerve and the nerve to stapedius, respectively. Parasympathetic nerve involvement can result in the reduction of secretory gland function. Eighty to eighty-five percent of patients make a full recovery within 3 months of the onset of symptoms. Recovery of some motor function in the first 5 to 7 days is the most favorable sign. A viral etiology (cause) is suspected but unproven.

2. Why did John have trouble contracting the muscles on the right side of his face and neck?

The muscles of facial expression are supplied by the branchial motor component of the facial nerve. A lesion to the right facial nerve anywhere along its course after it leaves the motor nucleus of VII (lower motor neuron lesion) would result in John's problems (see Lesion in Figure VII–6). The facial muscles insert into the skin. John tenses his facial muscles, including the platysma in the neck, for shaving. Paralysis of his facial nerve inactivated these muscles, which resulted in his shaving problems. The frontalis muscle elevates the eyebrow, and the orbicularis oculi muscle acts as a sphincter closing the eye. Loss of the right facial nerve would inactivate all of these muscles.

The facial nerve also supplies the orbicularis oris muscle that acts with its partner of the left side as a sphincter, closing the mouth. John's inability to close the right side of his mouth tightly caused him to dribble his soup. The facial distortion is due to the unopposed action of John's left facial muscles.

3. Why was John's mouth dry?

The facial nerve carries parasympathetic secretomotor fibers to the submandibular and sublingual glands as well as to the mucosa of the mouth. As John's mouth was dry, we know that the lesion to the facial nerve must have occurred before the parasympathetic component left the facial nerve as the chorda tympani. This would mean that, as well as branchial motor control loss, the secretomotor action of the facial nerve would also be lost and the production of saliva decreased (see Figures VII–1, Lesion B and VII–9).

4. What is the anatomic basis for the loss of taste to the anterior two-thirds of John's tongue on the right side?

Loss of taste to the anterior two-thirds of the tongue on the right side can result from a lesion of the right facial nerve anywhere along its course. To locate the specific site of the lesion, other deficits as well as the loss of taste must be identified.

For example, in John's case, because he has paralysis of all the muscles supplied by the facial nerve as well as the loss of secretion and taste to the anterior two-thirds of the tongue, the lesion must be in the facial canal before the branch to the pterygopalatine ganglion is given off.

5. How do substances in John's mouth give rise to electrical signals in gustatory neurons?

The four (or five) taste modalities are transduced by different types of receptor cells within the taste buds. The receptor cells are not evenly distributed; receptors for salt and sweet are most dense on the anterior parts of the tongue (predominantly cranial nerve VII), and the receptors for sour and bitter are most dense on the posterior parts of the tongue and epiglottis (predominantly cranial nerve IX).

Taste transduction involves gustatory receptor cells, which detect chemical compounds in the mouth and send signals to the primary gustatory (special sensory) neurons of cranial nerve VII and cranial nerve IX. The gustatory receptor cells are located in taste buds, which, in turn, are located in clusters on papillae on the dorsal surface of the tongue. The cells extend from the basal lamina to the mucosal surface where microvilli project from their apical tips into a depression (taste pore) on the papilla. Gustatory receptor cells, like olfactory receptor cells, are replicated throughout life.

Four taste modalities are well established: salt, sour, sweet, and bitter, and a fifth modality, umami (delicious taste) in response to some amino acids, is becoming increasingly recognized. Recent research has established that taste is transduced by two basically different mechanisms. One mechanism involves the direct interaction of taste stimuli with ion channels in the receptor cell membrane: salt (Figure VII–11A), sour, bitter, and possibly umami. The second mechanism involves the interaction of taste stimuli with membrane-bound receptors that activate one or more second-messenger pathways in the receptor cell: sweet (Figure VII–11B), bitter, and possibly umami. In both mechanisms, the intracellular Ca^{++} concentration increases, either by influx from the outside or release from intracellular stores, resulting in neurotransmitter release from the receptor cell. The released neurotransmitter(s) gives rise to trains of impulses in the primary gustatory neurons, which carry the information to the central nervous system.

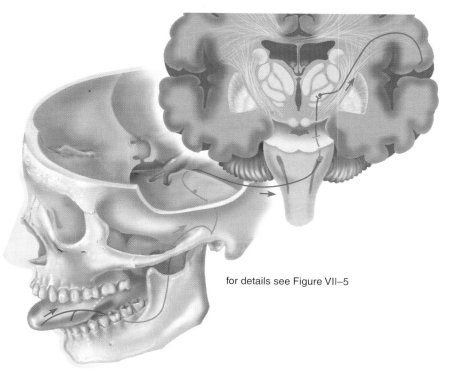

for details see Figure VII–5

SALT — direct pathway

SWEET — 2nd-messenger pathway

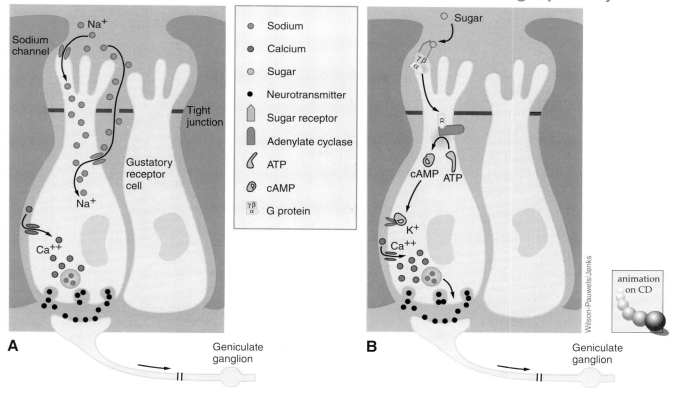

●	Sodium
●	Calcium
●	Sugar
●	Neurotransmitter
⬠	Sugar receptor
▮	Adenylate cyclase
⌇	ATP
⊘	cAMP
γβ/α	G protein

Na⁺

Sodium channel

Na⁺

Ca⁺⁺

Tight junction

Gustatory receptor cell

A

Geniculate ganglion

Sugar

cAMP ATP

K⁺

Ca⁺⁺

B

Geniculate ganglion

animation on CD

Wilson-Pauwels/Jenks

Figure VII–11 *A,* Na⁺ dissociates from NaCl (salt) in the mouth and flows into receptor cells through sodium channels. The resulting increase in intracellular positive charge activates voltage-gated Ca⁺⁺ channels, allowing Ca⁺⁺ influx and neurotransmitter release. *B,* Sugars bind to membrane-bound receptors, which associate with G proteins. The G protein releases its α subunit, which causes the production of cAMP. cAMP blocks K⁺ channels resulting in a depolarization of the receptor cell membrane, an influx of Ca⁺⁺, and neurotransmitter release. Na⁺ = sodium; NaCl = sodium chloride; Ca⁺⁺ = calcium; cAMP = cyclic adenosine monophosphate; K⁺ = potassium; ATP = adenosine triphosphate.

6. What is the anatomic basis of John's excessive tearing?

Because of the paralysis of his orbicularis oculi muscle, John cannot close his right eye and his right lower lid falls away from the conjunctiva. Therefore, his tears cannot be moved across his right eyeball to the lacrimal duct where they drain into his nose; as a result, his cornea drys out.

This has two consequences. Excessive tears collect in his right conjunctival sac and spill over onto his cheek (Figure VII–12). The dryness and irritation of his cornea, signaled by cranial nerve V_1 (part of the afferent limb of the blink reflex), stimulate the superior salivatory (lacrimal) nucleus, which, in turn, sends secretomotor signals via the greater petrosal nerve (cranial nerve VII) to the lacrimal gland to produce and release even more tears.

7. How does an understanding of John's excessive tearing problem help you to locate the site of the lesion?

The presence of tearing is helpful in the anatomic localization of the lesion. The parasympathetic fibers branch from cranial nerve VII at the geniculate ganglion and become the greater petrosal nerve. As a result, if a lesion is proximal to the geniculate ganglion, all modalities of cranial nerve VII, including tearing, will be lost. If

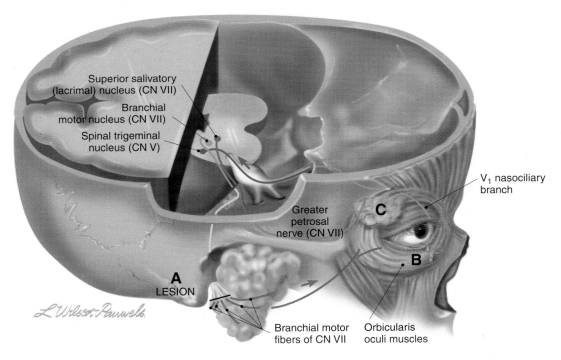

Figure VII–12 John's blink reflex is compromised due to *A*, lesion to the branchial motor fibers of cranial nerve VII. This causes *B*, tears to spill over the right conjunctival sac and *C*, stimulation of the lacrimal gland in response to the dry cornea.

the lesion is distal to the geniculate ganglion, all modalities of cranial nerve VII, except tearing, could be affected (see Figure VII–1, Lesion B). Because John does not have a dry eye due to loss of tearing, we know that his lesion must be located in the facial nerve distal to the geniculate ganglion.

8. Why was John's recovery so prolonged?

Unfortunately, John suffered from axonal damage to his facial nerve. Typically, in Bell's palsy there is no axonal damage. However, sometimes axonal loss does occur and there is electromyographic evidence of muscle degeneration in the face. In this case, recovery is prolonged because it is dependent on regeneration of the nerve, which may take years.

9. Why does John's right eye close every time he smiles?

After axonal damage of the right facial nerve, there may be regeneration with the risk of misdirection of the regenerating fibers. Aberrant reinnervation of facial muscles results in abnormal synkinesis (motor activity). For example, if some fibers from the motor neurons that initiate smiling regenerate and join with neurons innervating the orbicularis oculi, the result could be closure of the eye when the patient smiles spontaneously. Conversely, if some of the motor fibers that innervate orbicularis oris regenerate to join neurons that activate the labial muscles, the result could be a twitch of the mouth when the patient blinks.

In rare cases, the regenerating fibers originally supplying the submandibular and sublingual salivary glands aberrantly innervate the lacrimal gland via the greater petrosal nerve. This results in inappropriate unilateral lacrimation with eating. This condition is called "crocodile tears."

10. What other lesions could affect the motor component of the facial nerve?

A facial palsy can result from a lesion anywhere from the cortex to the site of innervation. Lesions are classified as (1) upper motor neuron lesions (UMNL) or (2) lower motor neuron lesions (LMNL).

Upper Motor Neuron Lesions

Cortical tumors, infarcts, and abscesses affecting upper motor neuron somata in the motor cortex, or its axon that projects to the facial nucleus, result in loss of voluntary control of only the lower muscles of facial expression contralateral to the lesion (Figure VII–13). Frontalis and orbicularis oculi muscles continue to function because the part of the facial nucleus that innervates them still receives input from the ipsilateral hemisphere (see Figure VII–7, expanded view of the nucleus). In many cases, however, there is preservation of emotionally motivated facial movements. This means that emotionally motivated input to the facial nucleus follows a different pathway than the corticobulbar output.

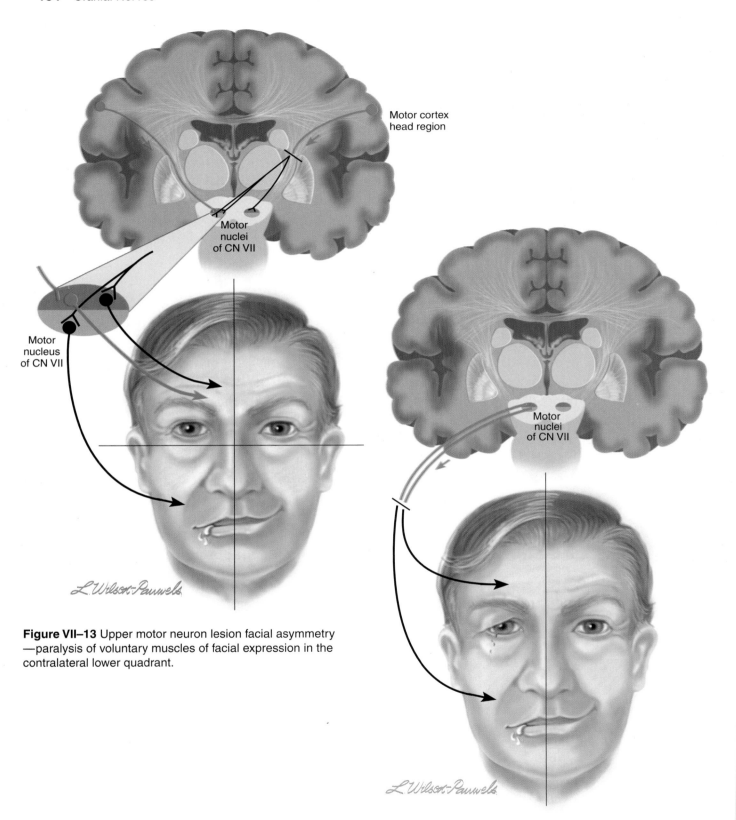

Motor cortex
head region

Motor
nuclei
of CN VII

Motor
nucleus
of CN VII

Figure VII–13 Upper motor neuron lesion facial asymmetry
—paralysis of voluntary muscles of facial expression in the
contralateral lower quadrant.

Motor
nuclei
of CN VII

Figure VII–14 Lower motor neuron lesion in Bell's palsy with facial
asymmetry—ipsilateral paralysis of upper and lower quadrants.

The most common UMNL that involves cranial nerve VII is a vascular infarct or stroke that damages neurons in the cortex or, more commonly, their axons in the internal capsule (see Figure VII–8, Lesion A). These axons may also be affected anywhere along their course.

Lower Motor Neuron Lesions

Lesions resulting from damage to the facial nucleus or its axons anywhere along the course of the nerve after it leaves the nucleus (Figure VII–14) are commonly called LMNL.

Lesions in the pons that involve the nucleus of cranial nerve VII are commonly due to an infarct involving the pontine branches of the basilar artery. This results in a complete paralysis of the facial nerve ipsilaterally, combined with motor weakness of the limbs on the contralateral side of the body due to damage of the descending corticospinal fibers from the motor cortex before they cross over in the medulla (see Figure VII–8, Lesion B). Such lesions often include paralysis of the lateral rectus muscle because the abducens nucleus is in close proximity to the facial nucleus (see Figures VII–3 and VII–7). Pontine tumors may also disrupt the facial nucleus and nearby structures.

As the nerve exits the brain stem it may be damaged by acoustic neuromas (see Chapter VIII, Figure VIII–12), meningiomas, and meningitis. Typically, cranial nerves VI, VIII, and sometimes V are also involved at this site. After entering the facial canal, the nerve is susceptible to fractures of the base of the skull, spread of infection from the middle ear, herpes zoster infections, and, as in John's case, idiopathic (unknown cause) inflammation (Bell's palsy). All the muscles supplied by the nerve are paralyzed ipsilateral to the lesion (see Figures VII–3 and VII–8, Lesion C). All actions of the facial muscles, whether motivated by voluntary, reflex, or emotional input, are affected and there is atrophy of the facial muscles. In an infant the mastoid process is not well developed, and the facial nerve is very close to the surface where it emerges from the stylomastoid foramen. Thus, in a difficult delivery, the nerve may be damaged by forceps.

CLINICAL TESTING

When testing cranial nerve VII, it is important to examine the five main functions (see also Cranial Nerves Examination on CD-ROM).

1. Function of the Muscles of Facial Expression

When examining the muscles of facial expression, the examiner should first observe the patient's facial movements when he is speaking. Next, the examiner should ask the patient to raise his eyebrows to assess the action of the frontalis muscle. Symmetric furrowing of the forehead indicates normal function (Figure VII–15A). Orbicularis oculi is tested by asking the patient to close his eyes as tightly as possible. This should

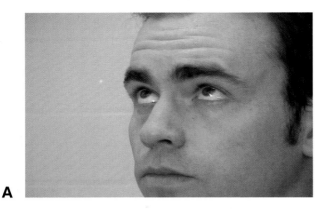

A

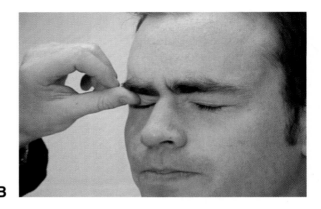

B

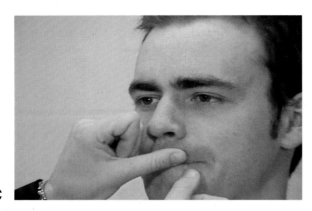

C

Figure VII–15 Clinical tests for the muscles of facial expression. *A*, Frontalis muscle. *B*, Orbicularis oculi muscle. *C*, Orbicularis oris muscle.

result in burrowing of the eyelashes and the examiner should be unable to open the patient's eyes when the patient resists (Figure VII–15B). The buccinator and orbicularis oris are tested by asking the patient to press the lips firmly together. If there is full strength, the examiner should be unable to separate the patient's lips (Figure VII–15C). The platysma can be tested by asking the patient to clench the jaw and the examiner should see the tightening of the muscle as it extends from the body of the mandible downward over the clavicle onto the anterior thoracic wall.

2. Taste from the Taste Buds

This is a special sensory nerve that carries taste sensation from the tongue in the chorda tympani to the nucleus solitarius via the nervus intermedius. This modality is assessed using a stick with a piece of cotton moistened in a sugary or salty solution. The patient is asked to protrude his tongue and the examiner touches his tongue on one side with the solution (Figure VII–16A). Before the patient returns his tongue into his mouth, he is asked to report what he tasted by pointing to the appropriate text on a sign, and then the examiner applies the solution to the other side of his tongue and asks the patient if there is any difference between the two sides (Figure VII–16B). The patient must rinse his mouth out with water before repeating the test with the next solution.

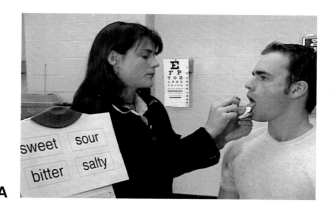 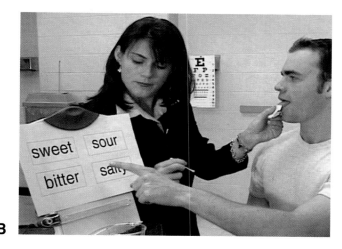

Figure VII–16 Clinical testing for taste. *A*, Four basic modalities (sweet, sour, bitter, and salty) are tested on each side of the tongue. *B*, The examiner holds the tongue and touches one side of it with a cotton swab soaked in a test solution while the patient points to the taste he perceives on the board. The examiner continues to hold the tongue so that the patient cannot close his mouth and distribute the test solution to other areas of the tongue.

3. Somatic Sensation from the External Ear

A sensory branch of cranial nerve VII supplies sensation to a small strip of skin on the posteromedial surface of the auricle, the skin of the concha, the wall of the external acoustic meatus, and the external surface of the tympanic membrane. Although sensation in this area can be tested by touching the skin with a sharp object for pain sensation and with cotton wool for light touch, abnormalities of sensation are rarely detected when this branch is involved.

4. Function of Stapedius Muscle

The stapedius muscle is responsible for dampening the oscillations of the ossicles of the middle ear. This muscle contracts reflexively to loud noises and at the onset of speech. Therefore, an individual who has damage to this branch of the nerve will hear noises louder on the affected side. This is referred to as hyperacusis. This can be assessed by standing behind the patient and suddenly clapping your hands together beside one ear and then the other ear and asking the patient if there is any difference in loudness between the two sides.

5. Secretomotor Innervation of the Lacrimal and Salivary Glands

The efferent fibers from the superior salivatory (lacrimal) nucleus travel in the nervus intermedius and divide into two nerves within the facial canal (see Figure VII–9). Tearing, which is a function of the lacrimal gland, can be tested using the Schirmer's test. One end of a piece of filter paper 5 mm wide and 25 mm long is inserted into the lower conjunctival sac, while the other end hangs over the edge of the lower lid. In a normal individual, the filter paper will absorb tears from the conjunctival sac and, after five minutes, have a moistened area that extends for approximately 15 mm along the filter paper. A moistened area of less than 10 mm is suggestive of hypolacrimia (underproduction of tears). For practical purposes this test is not commonly done. Direct questioning of the patient about the presence of dry eyes is adequate.

Although salivatory function cannot be tested easily at the bedside, it is still possible to assess it by asking whether the patient has a dry mouth and whether water is required to help with swallowing a meal.

ADDITIONAL RESOURCES

Adour KK, Ruboyianes JM, Von Doersten PG, et al. Bell's palsy treatment with acyclovir and prednisone compared with prednisone alone: a double-blind, randomized, controlled trial. Ann Otol Rhinol Laryngol 1996;105(5):371–8.

Bear MF, Connors BW, Paradiso MA. Neuroscience: exploring the brain. Baltimore: Williams & Wilkins; 1996. p. 190–8.

Brodal A. Neurological anatomy in relation to clinical medicine. 3rd ed. New York, Oxford: Oxford University Press; 1981. p. 495–503.

De Diego JI, Prim MP, De Sarria MJ, et al. Idiopathic facial paralysis: a randomized, prospective, and controlled study using single-dose prednisone versus acyclovir three times daily. Laryngoscope 1998;108(4 Pt 1):573–5.

Fitzerald MTJ. Neuroanatomy basic and clinical. 3rd ed. Toronto: W.B. Saunders Company Ltd.; 1996. p. 170–4.

Hanaway J, Woolsey TA, Mokhtar MH, Roberts MP Jr. The brain atlas. Bethesda, Maryland: Fitzgerald Science Press; 1998. p. 186–7.

Kandel ER, Schwartz JH, Jessell TM. Principles of neuroscience. 3rd ed. New York: Elsevier; 1991. p. 691.

Kiernan JA. Barr's the human nervous system. 7th ed. New York: Lippincott-Raven; 1998. p. 162–9.

Lindsay WK, Bone I, Callander R. Neurology and neurosurgery illustrated. 3rd ed. New York: Churchill Livingstone; 1997. p. 162–7.

MacLeish PR, Shepherd GM, Kinnamon SC, Santos-Sacci J. Sensory transduction. In: Zigmond MJ, Bloom FE, Landis SC, et al, editors. Fundamental neuroscience. San Diego: Academic Press; 1999. p. 671–717.

Moore KL, Dalley AF. Clinically oriented anatomy. 4th ed. New York: Lippincott, Williams & Wilkins; 1999. p. 862–4, 1083–5, 1097–101.

Nolte J. The human brain. 4th ed. Toronto: Mosby; 1999. p. 291, 301–4.

Noone J, Longe S. Bell's palsy in the primary care setting: a case study. Clin Excell Nurse Pract 1998;2(4):206–11.

Prim MP, De Diego JI, Sanz O. Prognostic factors in patients with idiopathic facial paralysis (Bell's palsy): a prospective study. J Otorhinolaryngol Relat Spec 1999;61(4):212–4.

Roob G, Fazekas F, Hartung HP. Peripheral facial palsy: etiology, diagnosis and treatment. Eur Neurol 1999;41(1):3–9.

Smith DV, Shepherd GM. Chemical senses: taste and olfaction. In: Zigmond MJ, Bloom FE, Landis SC, et al, editors. Fundamental neuroscience. San Diego: Academic Press; 1999. p. 719–59.

Young PA, Young JA. Basic clinical neuroanatomy. Philadelphia: Williams & Wilkins; 1997. p. 52, 291, 295.

VIII Vestibulocochlear Nerve

carries the special senses of hearing and balance

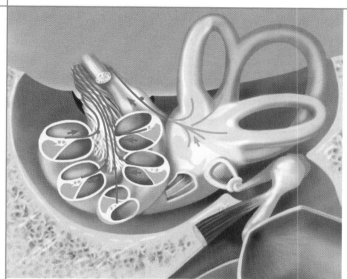

VIII Vestibulocochlear Nerve

CASE HISTORY

Paul, a 34-year-old sports reporter, noticed that he was having difficulty hearing in his right ear while talking on the telephone. Occasionally, he also heard ringing in his right ear, which had become progressively worse over the last couple of months. Paul racewalks in his spare time and lately has felt that his balance was off. One Sunday afternoon while on a training walk, Paul experienced a wave of vertigo (dizziness), lost his balance, and hit his head on a lamp post. He received a nasty cut to his scalp, so he went to the emergency department to get it sutured. He explained to the doctor that he was having some problems with his balance. When the physician examined Paul, she observed that he had abnormal eye movements. Although his eyes were able to move fully in all directions, he had horizontal nystagmus (see Clinical Testing in this chapter and in Chapter 13). His corneal reflexes, facial sensation, and facial movements were normal. When the physician examined Paul at the bedside, she found a marked reduction of hearing in his right ear. When a Weber's test was performed (see Clinical Testing in this chapter), Paul heard the ringing louder in his left ear. The remainder of his cranial nerves were functioning normally, but a full neurologic examination revealed that Paul had signs of cerebellar involvement. A magnetic resonance imaging (MRI) scan of his head was performed, and he was found to have a large tumor of his right eighth cranial nerve, which was pressing on his pons and cerebellum.

ANATOMY OF THE VESTIBULOCOCHLEAR NERVE

The vestibulocochlear nerve carries two types of special sensation: vestibular (balance) and auditory (hearing) (Table VIII–1 and Figure VIII–1). The sensory receptors of this nerve are situated in specialized areas on the inner walls of the membranous labyrinth. The membranous labyrinth is a delicate tubular structure filled with fluid (endolymph) lying inside a series of interconnected tunnels within the petrous temporal bone. The tunnels are referred to as the bony labyrinth.

The sensory transducers for both components of cranial nerve VIII are called hair cells (Figure VIII–2). The peripheral processes of the primary sensory neurons of the eighth cranial nerve extend for only a short distance from the bases of the hair cells in the vestibular apparatus and cochlea to the nerve cell bodies in the vestibular (Scarpa's) and spiral ganglia, respectively. The central processes of these neurons form the eighth cranial nerve, which travels through the internal auditory meatus in company with the seventh cranial nerve and enters the medulla at its junction with the pons. The central processes terminate within the vestibular and cochlear nuclei in the brain stem.

Table VIII–1 Nerve Fiber Modality and Function of the Vestibulocochlear Nerve

Nerve Fiber Modality	Nucleus	Function
Special sensory (afferent)	Vestibular	Balance
	Dorsal and ventral cochlear	Hearing

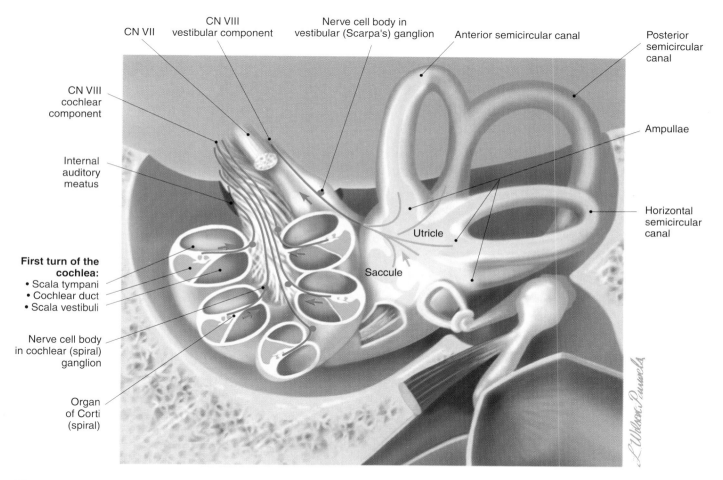

Figure VIII–1 Overview of the vestibulocochlear nerve, cranial nerve VIII. The membranous labyrinth (*blue*) contains endolymph.

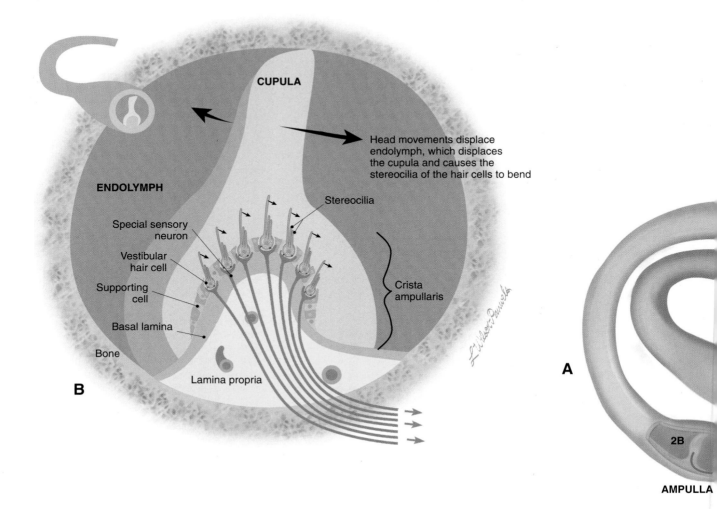

Head movements displace endolymph, which displaces the cupula and causes the stereocilia of the hair cells to bend

CUPULA

ENDOLYMPH

Special sensory neuron

Vestibular hair cell

Supporting cell

Basal lamina

Bone

Lamina propria

Stereocilia

Crista ampullaris

B

A

2B

AMPULLA

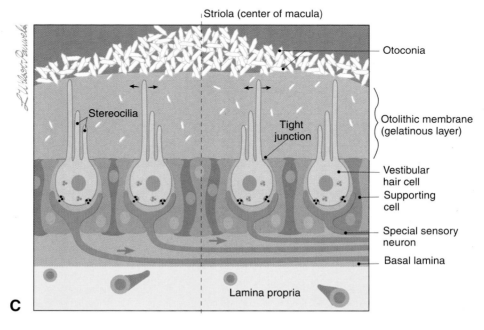

Striola (center of macula)

Otoconia

Stereocilia

Tight junction

Otolithic membrane (gelatinous layer)

Vestibular hair cell

Supporting cell

Special sensory neuron

Basal lamina

Lamina propria

C

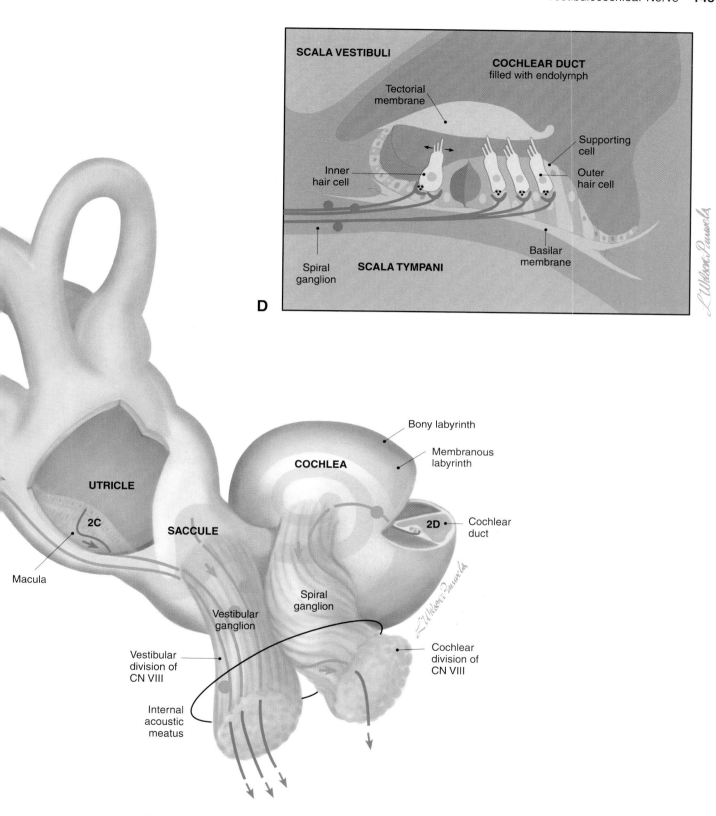

Figure VIII–2 *A*, Bony and membranous labyrinths of the vestibulocochlear nerve, cranial nerve VIII (removed from the surrounding petrous temporal bone). *B*, Ampulla of a semicircular duct (for clarity, structures are not drawn to scale). *C*, Macular hair cells of the utricle/saccule. *D*, The organ of Corti in the membranous labyrinth of the cochlear duct.

VESTIBULAR COMPONENT

The vestibular apparatus consists of the utricle, the saccule, and three semicircular canals. Hair cells, the sensory transducers, are located in specialized areas in the maculae in the utricle and saccule and the cristae in the semicircular canals.

Utricle and Saccule

The utricle and the saccule are expansions in the membranous labyrinth. Each contains a macula, which is a patch of hair cells overlain by a gelatinous sheet, called the otolithic membrane (from the Greek words *otos*, meaning ear, and *lithos*, meaning stone). The otolithic membrane includes millions of fine calcium carbonate particles, the otoconia, lying on its surface or embedded in its top layer (see Figure VIII–2C).

The main functions of the utricle and the saccule are to detect the position of the head and the movements of the head relative to gravity. As the head moves, the pull of gravity on the otolithic membrane causes it to lag behind. As the otolithic membrane shifts with respect to the underlying hair cells, the stereocilia of the hair cells are deflected. This deflection affects mechanically gated ion channels situated near the tips of the cilia (see Action Potentials in the Sensory Neurons, page 152). Depending on the direction of the deflection (see Figure VIII–2C), the cells will be either depolarized or hyperpolarized, resulting in an increase or decrease in the release of transmitter from the base and an increase or decrease in the generation of action potentials in the primary sensory neurons.

The hair cells of the maculae are oriented in all possible directions. Movement in a given direction will, therefore, excite some hair cells, inhibit others, and have little affect on still others. The macula of the utricle is oriented in the horizontal plane and the macula of the saccule lies in the vertical plane. Acceleration of the head in any direction deflects at least some hair bundles in both of these structures. As a result, the maculae of the utricle and saccule are able to send a complex signal to the brain encoding head movement.

> Because the maculae in the saccule and utricle respond to gravity, their function is severely compromised in space, under water, and under some conditions in an aircraft. In the absence of visual information, pilots are trained to trust the aircraft instruments rather than their own vestibular input.

Semicircular Canal

The three semicircular canals are tubes of membranous labyrinth extending from the utricle. They are oriented at right angles to each other (Figure VIII–3). Each canal has an expanded end, the ampulla, that contains a patch of hair cells similar to those in the utricle and saccule. The hair cells are covered by a gel-like structure, the cupula. Because the gel of the cupula does not contain otoconia, it does not respond to gravity. As the head moves, inertia causes the endolymph within the canals to lag behind and push on the cupula. As a result, the stereocilia of the ampullary hair cells bend, and the electrical properties of the hair cells change (see Figure VIII–2B). Working together, the hair cells send signals to the brain encoding head movement in all three planes.

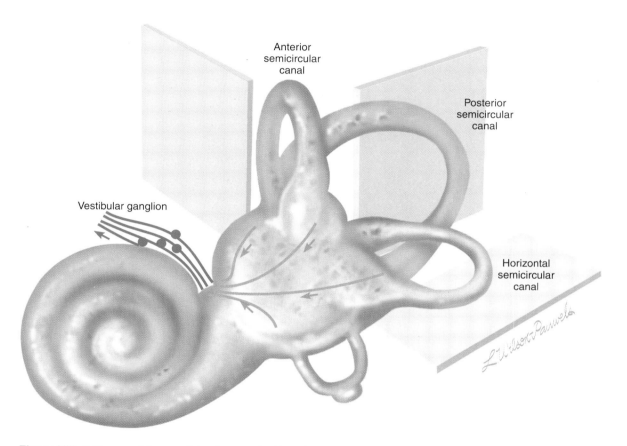

Figure VIII–3 Planes of the semicircular canals. Note that they are at right angles to each other.

Vestibular Nerve

Neurotransmitter released by the hair cells in the maculae and ampullae affects the peripheral processes of the primary sensory neurons whose cell bodies form the vestibular (Scarpa's) ganglion.

The central processes of the primary vestibular neurons form the vestibular component of the eighth cranial nerve. They travel with the cochlear afferents through the internal acoustic meatus to the vestibular nuclei at the junction of the pons and the medulla.

Vestibular Nuclear Complex

The vestibular nuclei integrate signals from the vestibular apparatus with sensory input from the spinal cord, cerebellum, and visual system and coordinate motor activities involved in eye and skeletal movements.

The vestibular nucleus (Figure VIII–4) is composed of four major subnuclei sitting in the floor of the medulla at the pontomedullary junction. They are named the superior, medial, lateral (Deiters'), and descending (inferior) nuclei.

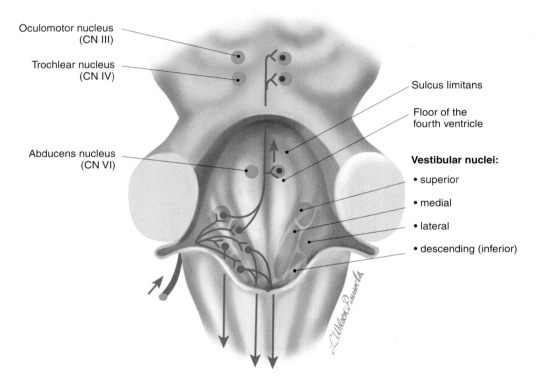

Figure VIII–4 Vestibular nuclear complex (posterior brain stem).

Input predominantly from the semicircular canals but also from the otolith organs projects to the

- *superior and medial nuclei,* which send signals in the contralateral ascending medial longitudinal fasciculus (MLF) to coordinate head and eye movements via cranial nerve nuclei III, IV, and VI (see Chapter 13). The medial nucleus also forms a substantial bilateral projection caudally to the cervical spinal cord via the descending MLF to coordinate postural head and neck movements (Figure VIII–5).

Input predominantly from the otolith organs but also from the semicircular canals projects to the

- *lateral (Dieters') nucleus,* which projects ipsilaterally to the spinal cord mostly in the lateral vestibulospinal tract (see below) to coordinate postural responses to gravity.
- *descending (inferior) nucleus,* which projects bilaterally to the cervical spinal cord by the descending MLF and to the vestibular parts of the cerebellum and the other vestibular nuclei (pathway not shown in Figure VIII–5).

All vestibular nuclei send a small number of axons via the thalamus to the somatosensory cortex, where they provide for conscious appreciation of balance and head position. Figure VIII–5 shows only the major projections from the nucleus.

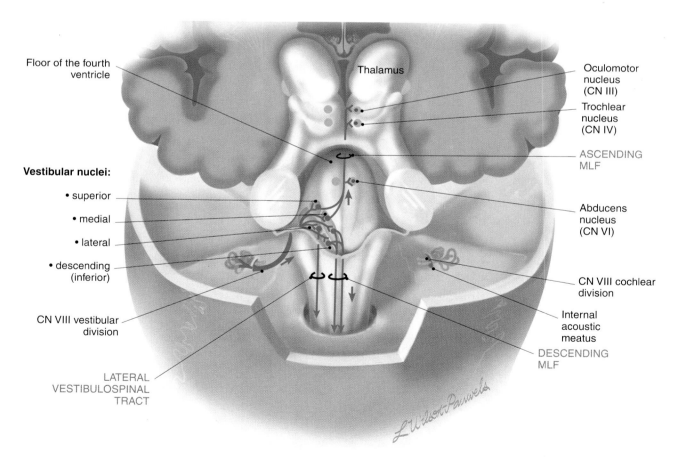

Figure VIII–5 Central afferent pathways of the vestibular division of the vestibulocochlear nerve. Note, the size of the brain stem is exaggerated. MLF = medial longitudinal fasciculus.

COCHLEAR COMPONENT

Sound waves in the air enter the external acoustic meatus and strike the tympanic membrane (ear drum), causing it to vibrate. The vibrations are carried through the middle ear cavity by a chain of three small bones, the malleus, incus, and stapes, to the oval window of the cochlea (Figure VIII–6). This chain of bones (ossicles) does more than simply transfer the force of the sound wave from the tympanic membrane to the oval window: it causes an amplification of the force per unit area applied to the oval window. This is brought about firstly by the fact that the tympanic membrane has an area that is approximately 15 times that of the oval window and secondly that the moving ossicles act as a system of levers, such that a given force at the tympanic membrane results in a much greater force at the stapes. As a result, about 60 percent of the sound energy applied to the tympanic membrane is transferred to the inner ear where it can cause movement of the fluid. If the ossicles were not present, more than 90 percent of the sound energy would be reflected back into the outer ear.

The cochlea, which comes from the Latin word meaning snail shell, is the spiral part of the bony labyrinth that houses the cochlear duct. The cochlea communicates with the middle ear cavity via two openings in the bone: the oval window (fenestra vestibuli), covered by the foot plate of the stapes, and the round window (fenestra cochlea), covered by a thin flexible diaphragm (the secondary tympanic membrane). Movements of the stapes in the oval window set up pressure waves within the perilymph, which travel through the cochlea and cause the round window diaphragm to vibrate. If the round window and its diaphragm were not present, movement of the stapes would be prevented by the incompressible nature of the fluid in the labyrinth. The round window, with its flexible diaphragm, allows the fluid to move slightly, allowing propagation of sound through the fluid.

The cochlear duct, part of the membranous labyrinth, divides the cochlea into three compartments (see Figure VIII–6, inset): the scala vestibuli, the scala tympani, and the cochlear duct itself (also known as the scala media). The part of the cochlear duct that is adjacent to the scala vestibuli is the vestibular (Reissner's) membrane, and the part that is adjacent to the scala tympani is the basilar membrane. The scalae vestibuli and tympani are continuous at the apex of the cochlea through an opening called the helicotrema. When the perilymph within the scalae vestibuli and tympani moves in response to sound, a responsive area of the basilar membrane oscillates, creating a corresponding disturbance in the the endolymph.

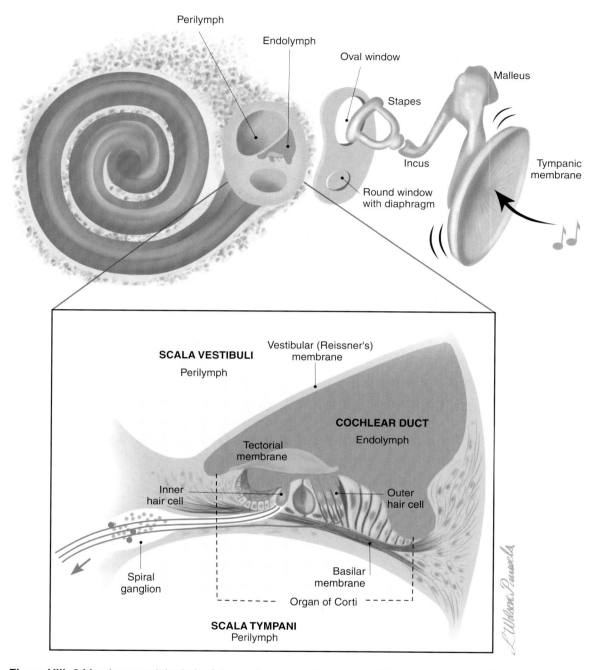

Figure VIII–6 Membranous labyrinth of the cochlear duct. The organ of Corti sits on the basilar membrane within the cochlear duct.

The organ of Corti sits on the basilar membrane. The hair cells in the organ of Corti are divided into two groups. The inner hair cells (3,500) form synaptic connections with more than 95 percent of the sensory afferents. They are primarily responsible for sound transduction. The stereocilia of the inner hair cells project into the endolymph within the cochlear duct. When the endolymph moves in response to movements of the basilar membrane, the cilia bend back and forth, opening and closing mechanically gated ion channels near their tips (Figure VIII–7). The resulting change in neurotransmitter release causes a corresponding change in the rate of impulse transmission along the auditory portion of the eighth nerve, which is interpreted as a change in the intensity of sound.

The outer hair cells, although they are much more numerous (12,000), form synaptic connections with only 5 percent of the primary afferents. Because of their unique ability to change their cell shape in response to electrical changes in their membranes, outer hair cells act to increase the movements of the basilar membrane and, therefore, to amplify the activity of the inner hair cells. This mechanism is called the cochlear amplifier.

Action Potentials in the Sensory Neurons

Transduction, that is the conversion of energy from mechanical to electrical forms, is accomplished by hair cells. Hair cells are flask-shaped or columnar cells of epithelial origin. A "hair bundle" of 20 to 300 stereocilia projects from the apical surface of each hair cell. The cilia vary in length and are arranged from shortest to longest. A filamentous protein, the tip link, connects the tip of one cilium to the side of the adjacent longer cilium (see Figure VIII–7). Mechanically gated ion channels are embedded in the membrane of the cilia near the attachment of the tip links. Deflection of the stereocilia toward the tallest of the stereocilia results in the opening of more ion channels. The composition of the endolymph in which the cilia are bathed is unlike any other extracellular fluid in that it has a high concentration of K^+ and is positively charged. Thus, on opening the mechanically gated channels, K^+ will flow from the extracellular environment into the cell, resulting in depolarization.

Hair cells store an excitatory neurotransmitter, probably glutamic acid, in synaptic vesicles at their bases, which is released tonically. Its rate of release increases or decreases as the ion channels open and close and the membrane depolarizes and hyperpolarizes. The released neurotransmitter binds with receptors on the peripheral processes of the primary sensory neurons. The change in neurotransmitter release causes a corresponding change in the rate of impulse transmission along the sensory neurons to the brain stem. The brain interprets increased and decreased impulse traffic as increased or decreased sound intensity.

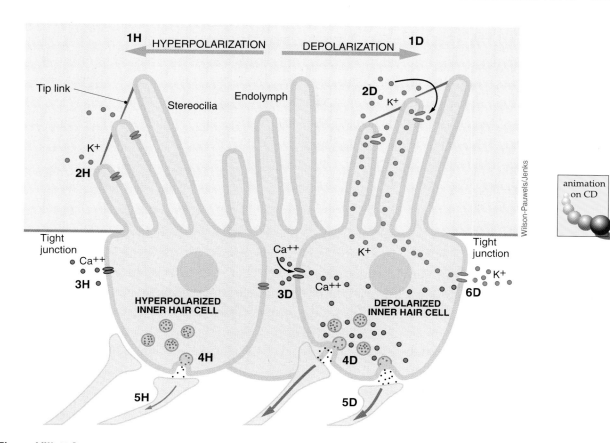

Figure VIII–7 Sensory transduction in an inner hair cell. Note that the size of the stereocilia relative to the body of the hair cell is grossly exaggerated for illustrative purposes. In reality, the maximum deflection of the stereocilia is ± 1 degree. At rest, approximately 15 percent of the ion channels are open. This allows an inward flow of cations, which are mainly K^+ because of their high concentration in the endolymph.

Depolarization (D)

1D Stereocilia are deflected toward the longest stereocilium.
2D Ion channels open, allowing increased entry of K^+ into the cytoplasm, depolarizing the cell.
3D Voltage-sensitive calcium channels open allowing the influx of Ca^{++}, which
4D enhances neurotransmitter release from synaptic vesicles.
5D As a result, impulse traffic along the primary afferents increases and the central nervous system interprets this as an increase in the sound intensity.
6D Excess K^+ is removed from the cell.

Hyperpolarization (H)

1H Stereocilia are deflected away from the longest stereocilium.
2H Ion channels close, decreasing the movement of K^+ into the cytoplasm, hyperpolarizing the cell.
3H Calcium entry into the cell decreases, which
4H decreases the release of neurotransmitter from synaptic vesicles.
5H As a result, impulse traffic along the primary afferents decreases, and the central nervous system interprets this as a decrease in sound intensity.

Pitch Discrimination

The structural features and mechanical properties of the basilar membrane vary along its length. At the base of the cochlea, the basilar membrane is short and tightly stretched across the base of the cochlear duct. High sound frequencies are required to set this area of the basilar membrane in motion. As one progresses along the cochlear duct from the base to the apex, the basilar membrane becomes wider and more relaxed, so that it responds to increasingly lower sound frequencies. As a result, sound at a given pitch will cause an area of maximal displacement at a particular position along the basilar membrane

The hair cells are situated along the length of the basilar membrane. A given hair cell will increase its firing rate only when the adjacent basilar membrane is vibrating. Therefore, activity in a given hair cell always signals the same pitch to the brain. Most sound in our environment is complex, that is, it consists of several tones at different pitches and intensities. Under normal circumstances, several areas of the basilar membrane, and therefore several groups of hair cells, are activated at once.

Central Pathways

In the auditory system, the sensory pathway from the periphery to the cerebral cortex is much more complex than in other sensory pathways. Primary sensory axons from the spiral ganglion project to the cochlear nucleus in the brain stem. The cochlear nucleus is located at the junction of the pons and medulla and is draped over the inferior cerebellar peduncle (Figure VIII–8). Functionally, it is divided into the dorsal and ventral cochlear nuclei.

Dorsal Cochlear Nucleus

- Neurons in the dorsal cochlear nucleus project across the midline via the dorsal acoustic stria and then rostrally in the lateral lemniscus to synapse in the contralateral inferior colliculus.

Ventral Cochlear Nucleus

- Neurons in the ventral cochlear nucleus project bilaterally via the trapezoid body (also known as the ventral acoustic stria) and the intermediate acoustic stria to the superior olivary nuclear complex for sound localization. Superior olivary nuclear complex neurons project via the lateral lemnisci to the inferior colliculi. The inferior colliculus projects in turn via the brachium of the inferior colliculus to the medial geniculate body of the thalamus and from here to the primary auditory cortex on the superior surface of the transverse temporal gyrus of the temporal lobe.

Because most of the projections from the cochlear nuclei are bilateral, unilateral lesions in the brain stem do not usually produce hearing deficits confined to one ear.

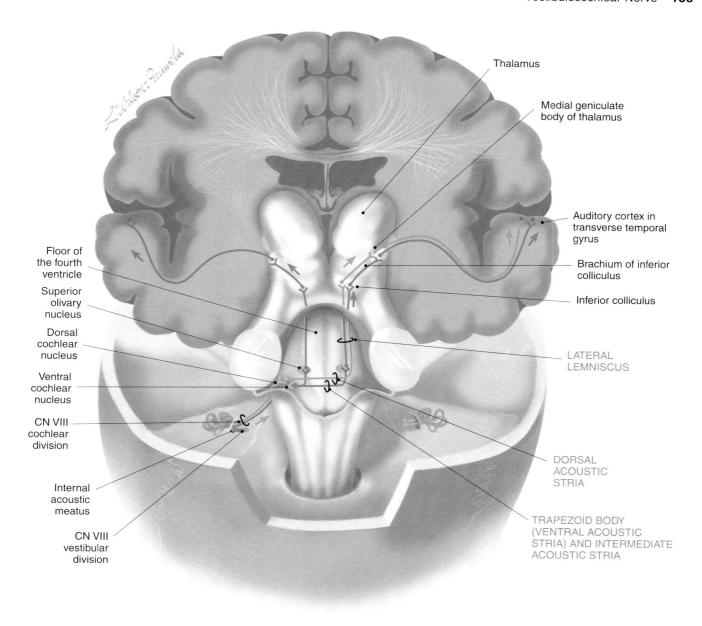

Figure VIII–8 Central afferent pathways of the cochlear division of the vestibulocochlear nerve. Note that the size of the brain stem is exaggerated. Only the major synapse points have been included.

Sound coming from one side of the head will arrive sooner, and its intensity will be slightly higher, in the ipsilateral ear. Cells in the superior olivary complex receive signals from both ears and therefore play a major role in the localization of sound. They compare the time of arrival (mainly for low frequency sounds) and intensity (mainly for high frequency sounds) and send this information to higher centers for sound localization. Humans can locate sound sources with an accuracy of a few degrees.

CASE HISTORY GUIDING QUESTIONS

1. What are other causes of hearing loss?

2. In cranial nerve VIII lesions, can there be impairment of vestibular function without hearing loss or vice versa?

3. What other cranial nerves can be involved when there is a tumor of cranial nerve VIII?

1. What are other causes of hearing loss?

Hearing loss can occur as a result of a lesion or disease process anywhere along the course of the auditory pathway from the auditory apparatus to the auditory cortex. The tympanic membrane, ossicles, and cochlea can be damaged by trauma or infection. Interference with the transmission of sound to the cochlea is defined as a **conductive** hearing loss. The organ of Corti and/or the auditory nerve may be damaged by noise exposure, infections, toxic drug exposure, or tumors. The central auditory pathways can be affected by strokes, multiple sclerosis, or tumors. Interference with the transduction mechanism or the transmission of impulses to the auditory cortex is defined as a **sensory** hearing loss. Damage to the transmission mechanism, transduction mechanism, or the auditory nerve results in hearing loss only on the affected side. Within the central nervous system, however, hearing signals are carried bilaterally in the lateral lemniscus and represented bilaterally in the auditory cortex. Unilateral lesions in the central nervous system, therefore, do not usually result in hearing loss in the ear on the affected side. In fact, total removal of one cerebral hemisphere of the brain in humans does not result in any major change of auditory sensitivity in either ear.

2. In cranial nerve VIII lesions, can there be impairment of vestibular function without hearing loss or vice versa?

Although referred to as the vestibulocochlear nerve, the nerve is actually two distinct nerves, vestibular and cochlear, that travel together. It is, therefore, possible for only one of the components to be involved in a disease process, but because of the close proximity in their peripheral course through the internal auditory meatus and across the cerebellopontine angle, both are usually involved simultaneously. Although Paul's tumor began on his auditory nerve, it expanded to involve the vestibular portion (Figure VIII–9) and eventually compressed his cerebellum.

Once the fibers enter the brain stem and synapse with their nuclei, the axons take different courses and are less likely to be affected simultaneously.

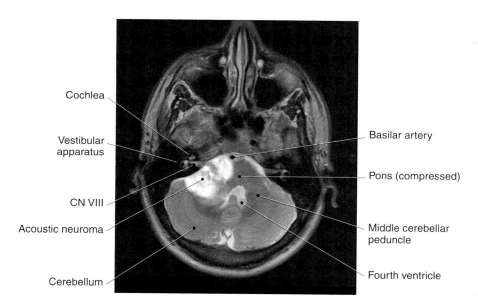

Figure VIII–9 Paul's magnetic resonance image showing a large acoustic neuroma on his right vestibulocochlear nerve (left side of the image). (Courtesy of Dr. D. S. Butcher.)

3. What other cranial nerves can be involved when there is a tumor of cranial nerve VIII?

Tumors such as neuromas and meningiomas typically compress cranial nerve VIII at the cerebellopontine angle. Other cranial nerve involvement is a reflection of the close proximity of these nerves to cranial nerve VIII. Cranial nerve VII is most often affected because it traverses the internal auditory meatus and the cerebellopontine angle beside cranial nerve VIII (Figure VIII–10). Facial nerve damage results in ipsilateral facial paralysis. Cranial nerve V can also be involved resulting in facial numbness, tingling, and sometimes facial pain. As the tumor enlarges it can also compress cranial nerves IX and X.

In addition to the peripheral cranial nerves, an expanding cerebellopontine angle tumor may compress the brain stem and interfere with transmission of sensory and motor signals between the cerebrum and spinal cord. Paul's MRI, Figure VIII–9, shows significant compression of his brain stem and cerebellum.

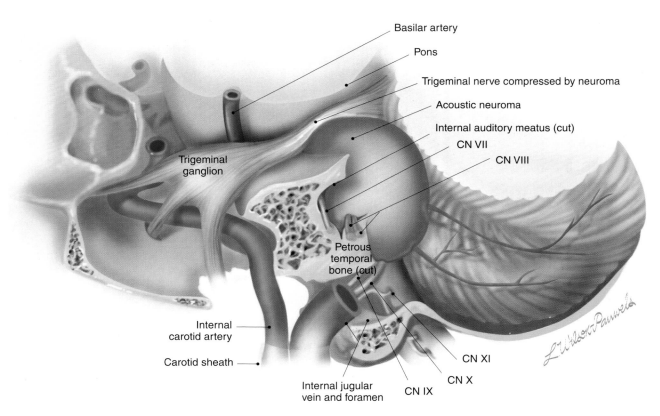

Figure VIII–10 An enlarged tumor (acoustic neuroma) in the cerebellopontine angle compromising cranial nerves V, VII, and the vestibular and cochlear divisions of VIII (*illustrated in green*). This is a sagittal section through the jugular foramen.

CLINICAL TESTING

Observation of the Vestibular Nerve

Because the vestibular nerve affects both eye and postural movements, the function of the nerve can be evaluated by observing the patient's eye movements and postural balance. As the emergency physician noted, Paul had horizontal nystagmus. Jerk nystagmus is the most common form and involves movements that alternate between a slow smooth phase and a fast (jerk) corrective phase. (See also Cranial Nerves Examination on CD-ROM.)

Nystagmus is always referred to in terms of the fast corrective phase. In other words, if the eyes appear to move slowly to the right with a quick corrective movement to the left, the patient has left nystagmus, regardless of the direction the patient is looking toward. When assessing the extraocular movements, the examiner should always look for evidence of nystagmus. The presence of inappropriate nystagmus can indicate pathology of the vestibular pathway in some circumstances; however, there are other causes of nystagmus that will not be addressed in this book.

Caloric Testing of the Vestibular Nerve

Integrity of the vestibular nerve and its end organs can also be assessed using caloric stimulation testing. This is not performed as a routine part of the bedside cranial nerve testing but is done if vestibular nerve impairment is suspected. Caloric testing involves irrigation of the external auditory canal with warm and cold water. The patient is tested with the head of the bed at 30° from the horizontal. This position brings the horizontal semicircular canals into a more vertical plane, which is a position of maximal sensitivity to thermal stimuli. Using cool water at 30°C, the external auditory canal is irrigated for 30 seconds. In a normal individual, the eyes tonically deviate to the irrigated side followed by nystagmus to the opposite side. The nystagmus appears after a latent period of about 20 seconds and persists for 1.5 to 2 minutes. The same procedure is repeated after approximately 5 minutes using warm water at 44°C. When warm water is used, nystagmus is toward the irrigated ear. These results can be summarized using the mnemonic COWS, Cold Opposite Warm Same. (See also Cranial Nerves Examination on CD-ROM.)

Simple Hearing Test for the Cochlear Nerve

Auditory stimuli (hearing) can be assessed easily at the bedside. The patient covers one ear and the examiner whispers into the patient's other ear and asks the patient to repeat what has been whispered. The examiner can increase the volume if the patient fails to hear. This is repeated on the other side and the two sides are compared.

If reduced hearing is detected, the next step is to determine whether this is due to a conductive or a sensorineural loss. Conductive loss implies an obstruction in the transmission of sound from the air to the cochlea. This could be due to wax, an ear infection, or could be caused by damage to the tympanic membrane or the ossicles. A sensorineural loss, on the other hand, implies damage to the auditory pathway anywhere from the cochlea to the auditory cortex. The two types of hearing loss can be distinguished by the use of the Rinne and Weber's tests. (See also Cranial Nerves Examination on CD-ROM.)

Rinne Test for the Cochlear Nerve

The Rinne test involves placement of a vibrating 512 Hz tuning fork on the mastoid process (Figure VIII–11). Sound from the tuning fork is carried to the cochlea via bone conduction, bypassing the middle ear amplification mechanism. When the patient can no longer hear the ringing sound, the fork is removed from the mastoid process and brought to within 2.5 cm of the external auditory meatus to permit air to conduct sound through the external and middle ear to the cochlea. A patient with normal hearing will be able to hear the tuning fork again. This constitutes a positive Rinne test. If an individual fails to hear the ringing when the fork is placed alongside the ear, this is a negative test and implies that there is a conductive defect with the problem located in the external or middle ear. (See also Cranial Nerves Examination on CD-ROM.)

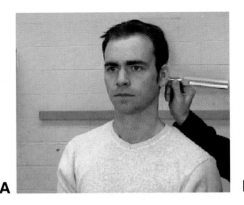 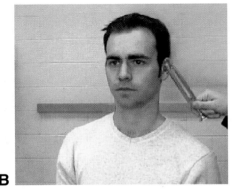

Figure VIII–11 The Rinne test to evaluate hearing. *A*, Vibrating tuning fork (512 Hz) is placed on the mastoid process. *B*, Tuning fork is brought to within 2.5 cm of the external auditory meatus. See text for further explanation.

Weber's Test

Weber's test can help distinguish between conductive deafness and sensorineural deafness. A vibrating 512 Hz tuning fork is placed in the middle of the forehead (Figure VIII–12). Sound is transmitted to the cochlea by bone conduction, bypassing the middle ear amplification system. In a person with normal hearing, the sound is heard equally in both ears. If an individual has sensorineural hearing loss, the ringing will not be as loud on the affected side. If an individual has a conductive hearing loss, the ringing will be louder on the affected side.

You can simulate a Weber's test on yourself. Hum a note. The sound from your larynx will be carried to your cochlea mainly by bone conduction. While humming, alternately block and unblock one external auditory meatus, creating a temporary conduction block. Note the change in perceived loudness in the blocked ear. (See also Cranial Nerves Examination on CD-ROM.)

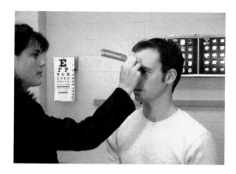

Figure VIII–12 Weber's test to distinguish between conductive and sensorineural deafness. A vibrating tuning fork (512 Hz) is placed in the middle of the forehead. See text for further explanation.

ADDITIONAL RESOURCES

Hackney CM, Furness DN, Benos DJ. Localisation of putative mechanoelectrical transducer channels in cochlear hair cells by immunoelectron microscopy. Scanning Electronmicrosc 1991;5:741–5.

Hackney CM, Furness DN, Benos DJ, et al. Putative immunolocalization of the mechanoelectrical transduction channels in mammalian cochlear hair cells. Proc Biol Sci 1992;248:215–21.

Hackney CM, Furness DN. Mechanotransduction in vertebrate hair cells: structure and function of the stereociliary bundle. Am J Physiol 1995;268(1 Pt 1):C1–13.

Hudspeth AJ. Hearing. In: Kandel ER, Schwartz JH, Jessell TM, editors. Principles of neural science. 4th ed. New York: McGraw-Hill; 2000. p. 590–612.

IX Glossopharyngeal Nerve

carries visceral and general sensation from the pharynx, carries subconscious sensation from the carotid sinus and body, and innervates the stylopharyngeus muscle and the parotid gland

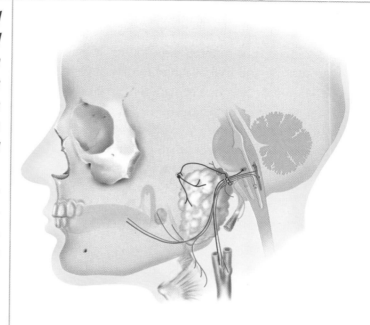

IX Glossopharyngeal Nerve

CASE HISTORY

Allen is a 43-year-old construction worker. While he was eating dinner, Allen developed pain in the left side of his throat. The pain was short, brief, and stabbing in nature and only occurred when he swallowed. Allen was eating fish at the time and assumed that a fish bone was lodged in his throat. He went to the emergency department and was assessed by an otolaryngologist, but nothing was found. It was assumed that a fish bone had scratched Allen's throat and that his symptoms would soon resolve.

A month later, Allen's pain was still present; in fact, it had increased. The pain occurred not only when he swallowed but also when he spoke and coughed. Again, while eating dinner, Allen experienced the same pain with swallowing. He got up from the table, but after a few steps he collapsed unconscious to the floor.

Although Allen quickly regained consciousness, he was immediately taken to the emergency department where he was put on a heart rate and blood pressure monitor to evaluate the function of his cardiovascular system. While he was on the monitor, the emergency room physician noticed an interesting correlation. Whenever Allen swallowed, he had a paroxysm (a sudden recurrence or intensification of symptoms) of pain followed invariably within 3 to 4 seconds by a decrease in heart rate (bradycardia) and a fall in blood pressure (hypotension). Allen was examined by a neurologist who noticed no evidence of reduced perception of pharyngeal pinprick or touch, or of pharyngeal motility. A diagnosis of glossopharyngeal neuralgia was made. Allen was treated with carbamazepine. His attacks of pain stopped and his cardiovascular function returned to normal.

ANATOMY OF THE GLOSSOPHARYNGEAL NERVE

The name of the glossopharyngeal nerve indicates its distribution (ie, to the glossus [tongue] and to the pharynx). Cranial nerve IX emerges from the medulla of the brain stem as the most rostral of a series of rootlets that emerge between the olive and the inferior cerebellar peduncle. The nerve leaves the cranial fossa through the jugular foramen along with cranial nerves X and XI (Figure IX–1). Two ganglia are situated on the nerve as it traverses the jugular foramen, the superior and inferior (petrosal) glossopharyngeal ganglia. The superior ganglion is small, has no branches, and is usually thought of as part of the inferior glossopharyngeal ganglion. The ganglia are composed of nerve cell bodies of sensory components of the nerve (Figure IX–2).

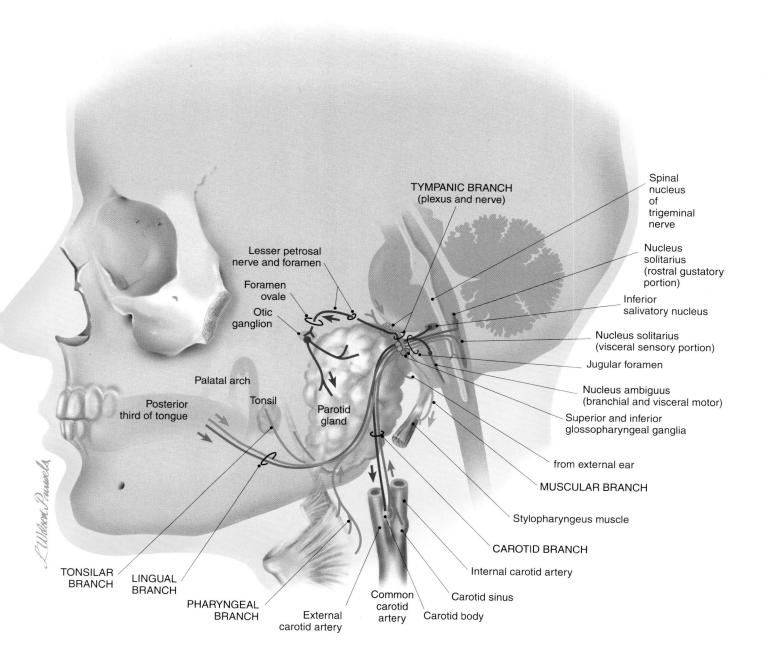

Figure IX–1 Overview of the glossopharyngeal nerve.

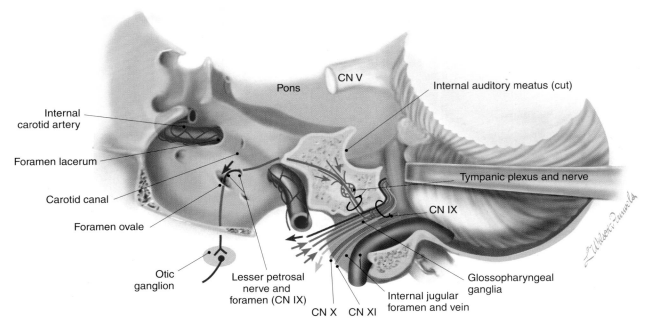

Figure IX–2 Tympanic branch of cranial nerve IX (cut through the petrous temporal bone).

As the nerve passes through the jugular foramen, it gives rise to six terminal branches. These are the tympanic, carotid, pharyngeal, tonsilar, lingual, and muscular branches (see Figure IX–1).

GENERAL SENSORY (AFFERENT) COMPONENT

The glossopharyngeal nerve carries general sensory signals from a small area of the external ear, tympanic cavity (see Figure IX–2), mastoid air cells, auditory tube, posterior third of the tongue, and entrance to the pharynx (Figure IX–3 and Table IX–1). The cell bodies of the sensory neurons are located in the inferior glossopharyngeal ganglion, and their axons contribute to the tympanic, pharyngeal, lingual, and tonsilar branches. The tympanic branch is formed by the union of the tympanic plexus axons and comprises general sensory and visceral motor fibers. The sensory fibers descend through the tiny tympanic canaliculus and join the main trunk of the glossopharyngeal nerve at its inferior ganglion (see Figure IX–2). Sensation from the pharynx, including the soft palate, tonsil, and the posterior third of the tongue, is carried in the pharyngeal, tonsilar, and lingual branches.

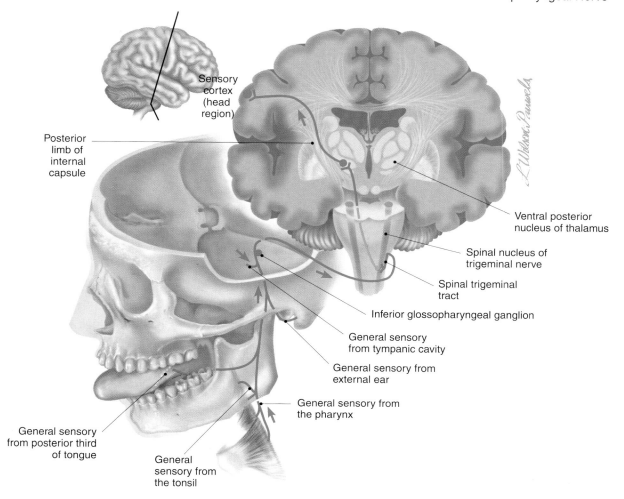

Figure IX–3 General sensory component of the glossopharyngeal nerve.

Table IX–1 Nerve Fiber Modality and Function of the Glossopharyngeal Nerve

Nerve Fiber Modality	Nucleus	Function
General sensory (afferent)	Spinal trigeminal	Provides general sensation from the posterior one-third of the tongue, the tonsil, the skin of the external ear, the internal surface of the tympanic membrane, and the pharynx
Visceral sensory (afferent)	Of the tractus solitarius—middle part	Provides subconscious sensation from the carotid body (chemoreceptors) and from the carotid sinus (baroreceptors)
Special sensory (afferent)	Of the tractus solitarius—rostral part (gustatory nucleus)	Carries taste from the posterior one-third of the tongue
Branchial motor (efferent)	Ambiguus	Supplies the stylopharyngeus muscle
Visceral motor (parasympathetic efferent)	Inferior salivatory Ambiguus	Stimulates the parotid gland For control of blood vessels in the carotid body

The central processes for pain enter the medulla and descend in the spinal trigeminal tract to end on the caudal part of the spinal nucleus of the trigeminal nerve (Figure IX–4). From the nucleus, processes of secondary neurons cross the midline in the medulla and ascend to the contralateral ventral posterior nucleus of the thalamus. From the thalamus, processes of tertiary neurons project to the post-central sensory gyrus (head region) (see Figure IX–3). The same pathway is suspected for touch and pressure and is important in the "gag" reflex (see Case History Guiding Questions, #7). These sensations operate at a "conscious" level of awareness.

VISCERAL SENSORY (AFFERENT) COMPONENT

Visceral sensory fibers operate at a "subconscious" level of awareness. Chemoreceptors in the carotid body monitor oxygen (O_2), carbon dioxide (CO_2), and acidity/alkalinity (pH) levels in circulating blood and baroreceptors (stretch receptors) in the carotid sinus monitor arterial blood pressure. These sensations are relayed in the carotid branch of the glossopharyngeal nerve (Figure IX–5) to the inferior glossopharyngeal ganglion where the nerve cell bodies are located. From these neurons, central processes pass to the tractus solitarius to synapse with nucleus solitarius cells in the middle third of the nucleus (see Figure IX–4). From this nucleus, connections

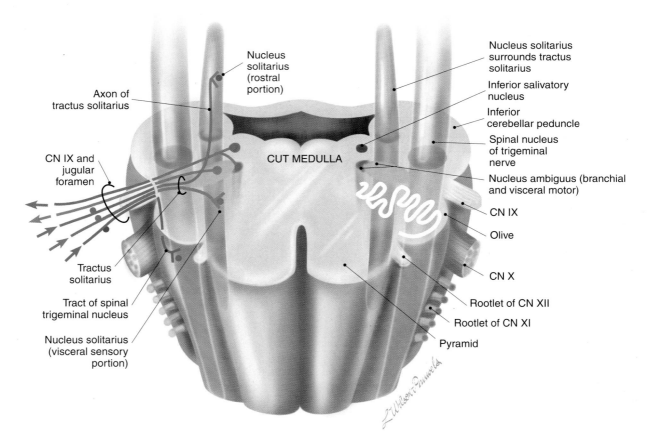

Figure IX–4 Cross-section of the medulla at the point of entry of cranial nerve IX illustrating the nuclei associated with this nerve.

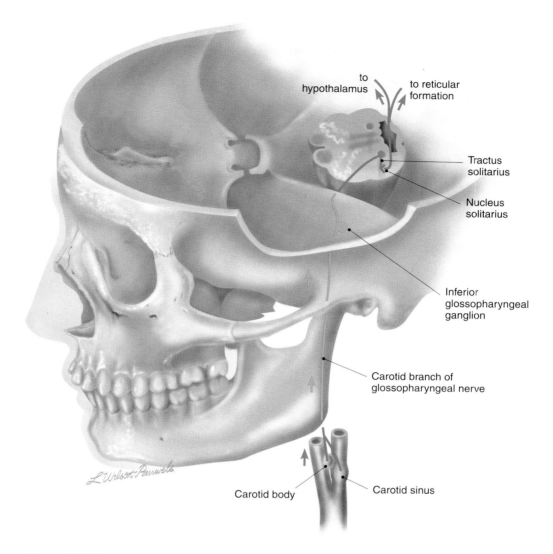

Figure IX–5 Visceral sensory component of the glossopharyngeal nerve—elevated brain stem.

are made with the reticular formation and the hypothalamus for the appropriate reflex responses for the control of respiration, blood pressure, and cardiac output.

Carotid Body

The carotid body is a small (3 mm × 6 mm in diameter) chemoreceptor organ located at the bifurcation of the carotid artery (see Figures IX–5 and IX–6). Very low levels of O_2, high levels of CO_2, and lowered pH levels (increased acidity) in the blood all cause an increase in the frequency of sensory signal traffic in the carotid branch of the glossopharyngeal nerve.

The transduction mechanism is not well understood. Glomus cells excite or inhibit sensory nerve endings in response to changing conditions in the blood. In return, the nerve endings may alter the function of the glomus cells, possibly in a way that changes their sensitivity to O_2, CO_2, and pH.

The carotid body is supplied by a plexus of autonomic efferent nerves; sympathetic nerves traveling with the blood vessels and glossopharyngeal and vagal parasympathetic nerves. Their role in carotid body function is unknown.

Carotid Sinus

The carotid sinus is a dilatation of the internal carotid artery at its origin off the common carotid artery and may extend into the proximal part of the internal carotid artery. It responds to changes in arterial blood pressure. The walls of the sinus are characterized by having a thinner tunica media and a relatively thick tunica adventitia. The adventitia contains many sensory nerve endings (stretch receptors) of the glossopharyngeal nerve that respond to increases in blood pressure within the sinus by initiating impulses that reflexively lower the pressure (see Figure IX–6).

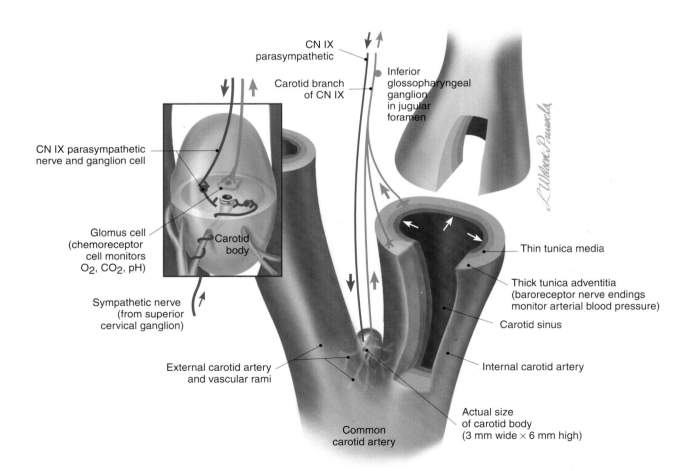

Figure IX–6 The bifurcation of the common carotid artery demonstrating baroreceptors in the wall of the carotid sinus and chemoreceptors within the carotid body.

SPECIAL SENSORY (AFFERENT) COMPONENT

Taste sensation from the posterior one-third of the tongue (predominantly sour and bitter), including the vallate papillae, is carried by special sensory axons toward their cell bodies in the inferior glossopharyngeal ganglion. Central processes from these neurons pass through the jugular foramen, enter the medulla, and ascend in the tractus solitarius to synapse in the rostral part of the nucleus solitarius (gustatory nucleus) (Figure IX–7). Axons of cells in the nucleus solitarius then ascend in the central tegmental tract of the brain stem to reach the ipsilateral ventral posterior nucleus of the thalamus (some studies show bilateral projections but more recent studies indicate that the projection is ipsilateral). From the thalamus, fibers ascend

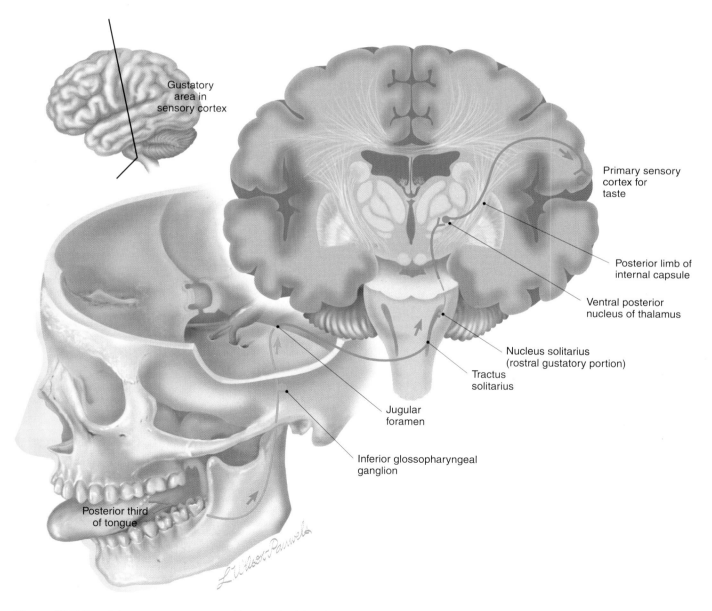

Figure IX–7 Special sensory component (for taste) of the glossopharyngeal nerve.

through the posterior limb of the internal capsule to reach the primary sensory cortex in the inferior third of the postcentral gyrus where taste is perceived. See Chapter VII for a description of sensory transduction in the taste buds.

BRANCHIAL MOTOR (EFFERENT) COMPONENT

In response to information received from the premotor sensory association cortex and other cortical areas, upper motor neurons in the primary motor cortex send impulses via corticobulbar fibers through the internal capsule and through the basis pedunculi to synapse bilaterally on the lower motor neurons in the rostral part of the nucleus ambiguus (Figures IX–8 and IX–9). The axons of these lower motor neurons join the other modalities of cranial nerve IX to emerge as three or four rootlets in the groove between the olive and the inferior cerebellar peduncle just rostral to the rootlets of the vagus nerve (see Figure IX–8). The glossopharyngeal nerve then passes laterally in the posterior cranial fossa to leave the skull through the jugular foramen just anterior to the vagus and accessory nerves. The branchial motor axons branch off as a muscular branch that descends in the neck deep to the styloid process of the sphenoid bone, curves forward around the posterior border of the stylopharyngeus muscle, and enters it to innervate its muscle fibers. The stylopharyngeus muscle elevates the pharynx during swallowing and speech (see Figure IX–9).

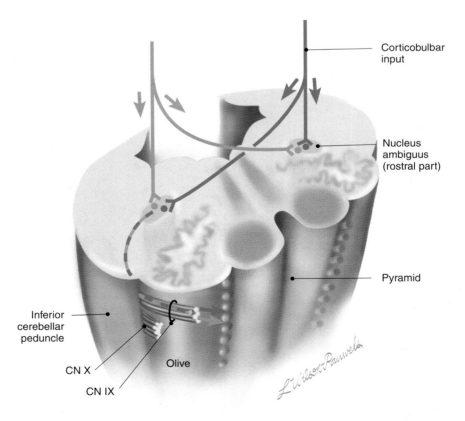

Figure IX–8 Branchial motor component of the glossopharyngeal nerve (section through the cranial part of the medulla).

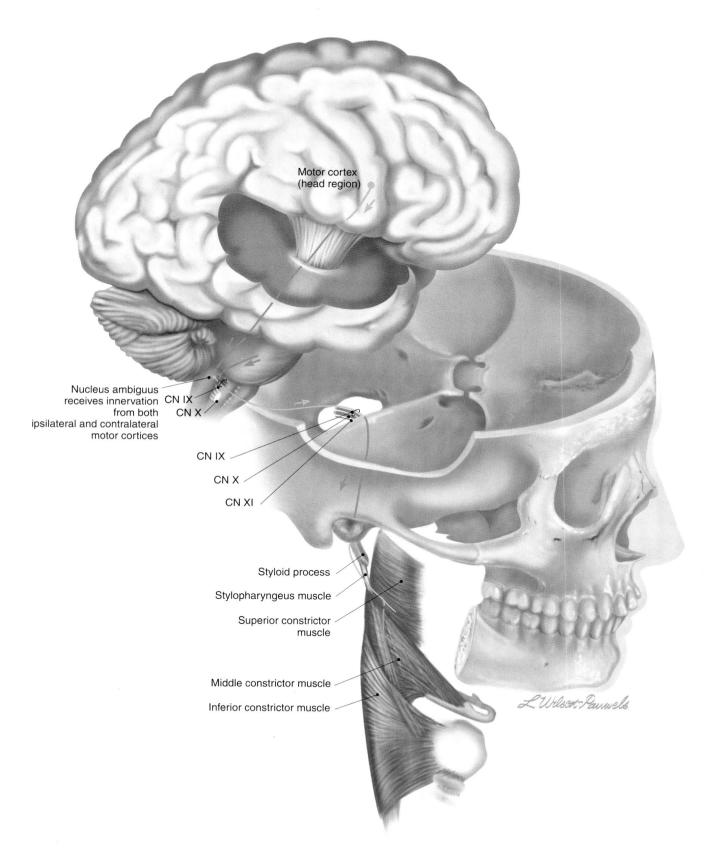

Motor cortex
(head region)

Nucleus ambiguus
receives innervation
from both
ipsilateral and contralateral
motor cortices

CN IX

CN X

CN IX

CN X

CN XI

Styloid process

Stylopharyngeus muscle

Superior constrictor
muscle

Middle constrictor muscle

Inferior constrictor muscle

Figure IX–9 Branchial motor component of the glossopharyngeal nerve.

VISCERAL MOTOR
(PARASYMPATHETIC EFFERENT) COMPONENT

Preganglionic neurons of the parasympathetic motor fibers are located in the inferior salivatory nucleus (see Figure IX–4) in the medulla. These neurons are influenced by stimuli from the hypothalamus (eg, dry mouth in response to fear) and the olfactory system (eg, salivation in response to smelling food). Axons from the inferior salivatory nucleus join the other components of cranial nerve IX in the medulla and travel with them into the jugular foramen (Figure IX–10). At the inferior ganglion, the visceral motor fibers leave the other modalities of cranial nerve IX as a component of the tympanic branch. They ascend to traverse the tympanic canaliculus and enter the tympanic cavity. Here they pass along the tympanic plexus on the surface of the promontory of the middle ear cavity. From the tympanic plexus, the visceral motor fibers form the lesser petrosal nerve that goes through a small canal back into the cranium to reach the internal surface of the temporal bone in the middle cranial fossa. The nerve emerges through a small opening, the lesser petrosal foramen, lateral to the foramen for the greater petrosal nerve (see Figure IX–10). The lesser petrosal nerve then passes forward to descend through the foramen ovale to synapse in the otic ganglion that usually surrounds the nerve to the medial pterygoid muscle, a branch of V_3. From the otic ganglion, postganglionic fibers join the auriculotemporal nerve (a branch of V_3) to supply secretomotor fibers to the parotid gland (Figure IX–11). Sympathetic nerves reach the parotid gland from the sympathetic plexus surrounding the external carotid artery and its branches in the area.

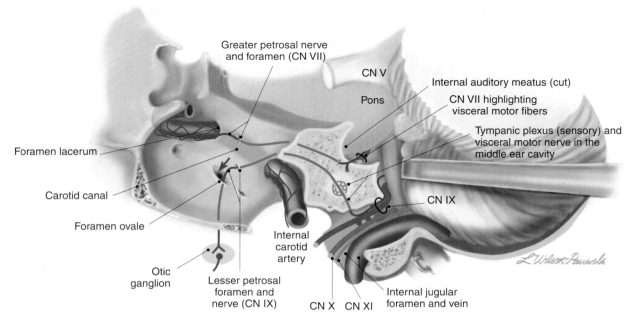

Figure IX–10 Lesser petrosal nerve (visceral motor IX) and greater petrosal nerve (visceral motor VII) and surrounding structures (sagittal section through the jugular foramen showing cut petrous temporal bone).

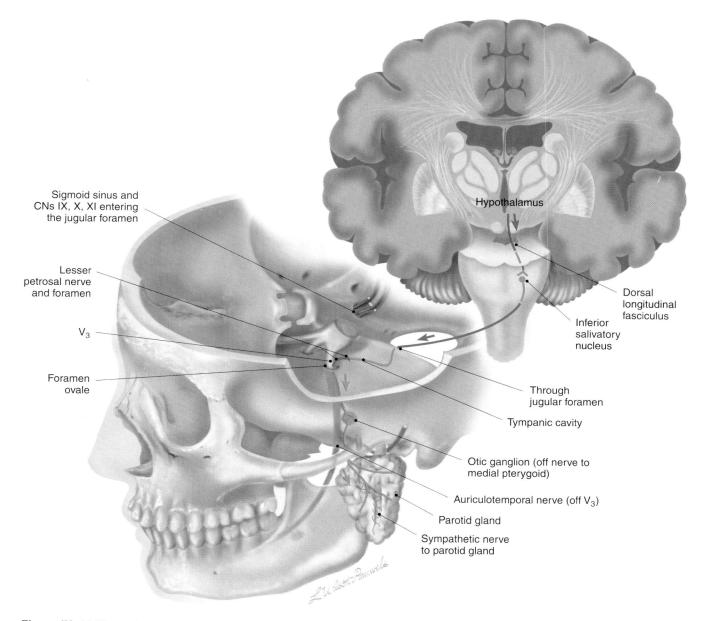

Sigmoid sinus and
CNs IX, X, XI entering
the jugular foramen

Lesser
petrosal nerve
and foramen

V₃

Foramen
ovale

Hypothalamus

Dorsal
longitudinal
fasciculus

Inferior
salivatory
nucleus

Through
jugular foramen

Tympanic cavity

Otic ganglion (off nerve to
medial pterygoid)

Auriculotemporal nerve (off V₃)

Parotid gland

Sympathetic nerve
to parotid gland

Figure IX–11 Visceral motor component of the glossopharyngeal nerve.

CASE HISTORY GUIDING QUESTIONS

1. What is glossopharyngeal neuralgia?
2. What is the cause of glossopharyngeal neuralgia?
3. What is allodynia?
4. Why did swallowing cause Allen pain?
5. Why did Allen collapse on the floor?
6. Why was carbamazepine used to treat Allen?
7. What is the gag reflex, and why don't we gag every time a bolus of food passes through the pharynx?

1. What is glossopharyngeal neuralgia?

Glossopharyngeal neuralgia* is characterized by severe, sharp, lancinating pain in the region of the tonsil, radiating to the ear. It is similar to trigeminal neuralgia (see Chapter V) in its timing and its ability to be triggered by various stimuli. For example, pain may be initiated by yawning, swallowing, or contact with food in the tonsilar region. In rare instances, the pain may be associated with syncope (a fall in heart rate and blood pressure resulting in fainting).

2. What is the cause of glossopharyngeal neuralgia?

Typically, glossopharyngeal neuralgia is idiopathic; that is, no cause can be identified. Occasionally glossopharyngeal neuralgia is secondary to the compression of cranial nerve IX by carotid aneurysms, oropharyngeal malignancies, peritonsillar infections, or lesions at the base of the skull.

3. What is allodynia?

Allodynia is pain that results from a touch stimulus that normally would not cause pain. The pain is usually burning or lancinating in quality.

4. Why did swallowing cause Allen pain?

Sensory nerve endings in the mucosa of Allen's pharynx were stimulated by the passage of a bolus of food and by the movements of the underlying muscles involved

---

*Some authors use the term vagoglossopharyngeal neuralgia or glossopharyngeal and vagal neuralgia, instead of glossopharyngeal neuralgia, implying that the pain can radiate into the distribution of the vagus nerve as well as that of the glossopharyngeal nerve. However, the original term, glossopharyngeal neuralgia, is recognized by most neurologists and is more commonly used.

in swallowing, coughing, and speaking. These usually harmless stimuli set off a barrage of pain impulses within the nervous system.

5. Why did Allen collapse on the floor?

Allen collapsed on the floor because his blood pressure dropped so low that he could not maintain adequate blood flow to his brain. The mechanism for Allen's fall in blood pressure and heart rate is not well understood. One hypothesis is that when the pain is most intense, general sensory impulses from the pharynx stimulate the nucleus of the tractus solitarius, which, in turn, stimulates vagal nuclei. Impulses from the parasympathetic component of the vagus nerve act to slow the heart rate and decrease blood pressure.

Alternatively, the rapidly firing general sensory afferents may, through ephaptic transmission,* give rise to action potentials in the visceral afferent axons from the carotid sinus as they travel together in the main trunk of the glossopharyngeal nerve. The carotid nerve would then falsley report increased blood pressure, causing a reflexive decrease in heart rate and blood pressure via connections in the brain stem.

6. Why was carbamazepine used to treat Allen?

Carbamazepine is a sodium channel blocking drug that is used to treat a wide range of conditions from seizures to neuropathic pain. Carbamazepine reduces the neuron's ability to fire trains of action potentials at high frequency and therefore shortens the duration of the paroxysm and frequently abolishes the attacks.

7. What is the gag reflex, and why don't we gag every time a bolus of food passes through the pharynx?

The gag is a protective reflex that prevents the entry of foreign objects into the alimentary and respiratory passages. A touch stimulus to the back of the tongue or pharyngeal walls elicits the gag (see Clinical Testing). Since the passage of a bolus of food through the pharynx stimulates the tongue and pharyngeal walls, we have to ask why swallowing does not elicit a gag reflex.

Although the exact mechanism is not well understood, it is generally accepted that when a swallowing sequence is initiated, probably by signals from the cerebral cortex to swallowing center(s) in the brain stem, simultaneous inhibitory signals are sent to the gag center in the brain stem to turn off the gag reflex.

---

*Ephaptic transmission occurs when a rapidly firing nerve changes the ionic environment of adjacent nerves sufficiently to give rise to action potentials in them. These "artificial synapses" often result from a breakdown in myelin.

A gag is not a partial vomit. Four events occur in the gag reflex (Figure IX–12):

A. An irritant is sensed in the mouth.

B. The soft palate elevates and is held firmly against the posterior pharyngeal wall closing off the upper respiratory airway.

C. The glottis is closed to protect the lower respiratory passages.

D. The pharynx is constricted to prevent entry into the alimentary tract, the pharyngeal wall constricts, and the tongue moves the contents of the pharynx forward to expel the offending foreign object from the mouth.

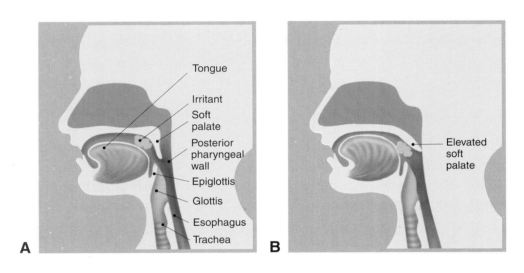
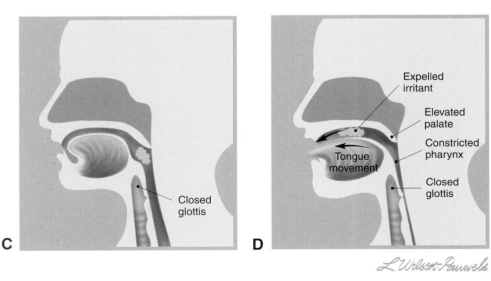

Figure IX–12 Steps in the gag reflex. *A*, Irritant in the mouth. *B*, Soft palate elevates, closing the upper respiratory airway. *C*, Glottis is closed to protect the lower respiratory airway. *D*, Pharyngeal wall constricts causing expulsion of the foreign object.

The sensitivity of the gag reflex can be affected by cortical events. It can be suppressed almost completely or enhanced such that even brushing the teeth or the sight of a dental impression tray can lead to gagging.

CLINICAL TESTING

Although cranial nerve IX comprises general sensory and motor, visceral sensory and motor, and special sensory components, from a practical point of view only the general sensory component is tested at the bedside. Clinically, cranial nerves IX and X are assessed by testing the gag reflex. The gag reflex involves both cranial nerves—the glossopharyngeal being the sensory afferent input and the vagus carrying the motor efferents. When assessing the gag reflex, right and left sides of the pharynx should be lightly touched with a tongue depressor (Figure IX–13). The sensory limb of the reflex is considered to be intact if the pharyngeal wall can be seen to contract after each side has been touched. (See also Cranial Nerves Examination on CD-ROM.)

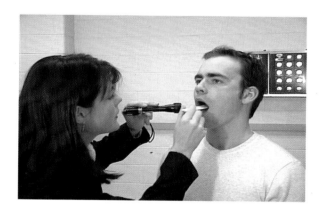

Figure IX–13 Testing the gag reflex by lightly touching the wall of the pharynx.

ADDITIONAL RESOURCES

Brodal A. Neurological anatomy in relation to clinical medicine. 3rd ed. New York: Oxford University Press; 1981. p.460–4, 467.

Ceylan S, Karakus A, Duru S, et al. Glossopharyngeal neuralgia: a study of 6 cases. Neurosurg Rev 1997;20(3):1996–2000.

Dalessio DJ. Diagnosis and treatment of cranial neuralgias. Med Clin North Am 1991;75(3):605–15.

Dubner R, Sessle BJ, Storey AT. The neural basis of oral and facial function. New York: Plenum Press; 1978. p. 370–2.

Eyzaguirre C, Abudara V. Carotid body glomus cells; chemical secretion and transmission (modulation?) across cell-nerve ending junctions. Respir Physiol 1999;115:135–49.

Fitzerald MTJ. Neuroanatomy basic and clinical. 3rd ed. Toronto: W.B. Saunders Company, Ltd.; 1996. p.147–50, 190–1.

Glossopharyngeal neuralgia with cardiac syncope: treatment with a permanent cardiac pacemaker and carbamazepine. Arch Intern Med 1976;136:843–5.

Haines DE. Fundamental neuroscience. New York: Churchill Livingstone; 1997. p. 261.

Hanaway J, Woolsey TA, Mokhtar MH, Roberts MP Jr. The brain atlas. Bethesda (MD): Fitzgerald Science Press, Inc.; 1998. p. 180–1, 186–7, 194–5.

Kandel ER, Schwartz JH, Jessel TM. Principles of neuroscience. 3rd ed. New York: Elsevier Science Inc.; 1996. p. 770–2.

Kiernan JA. Barr's the human nervous system. 7th ed. New York: Lippincott-Raven; 1998. p. 169–74.

Kong Y, Heyman A, Entman ML, McIntosh HD. Glossopharyngeal neuralgia associated with bradycardia, syncope, and seizures. Circulation 1964;30:109–12.

Loewy AD, Spyer KM. Central regulation of autonomic functions. New York: Oxford University Press; 1990. p. 182–4.

Miller AJ. The neuroscientific principles of swallowing and dysphagia. San Diego: Singular Publishing Group, Inc.; 1999. p. 100–1.

Moore KL, Dalley AF. Clinically oriented anatomy. 4th ed. New York: Lippincott Williams & Wilkins; 1999. p. 1104–5.

Nolte J. The human brain. 4th ed. Toronto: Mosby Inc.; 1999. p. 288, 305.

Verna A. The mammalian carotid body: morphological data. In: Gonzalez C, editor. The carotid body chemoreceptors. Austin (TX): Chapman & Hall, Landes Bioscience; 1997. p. 1–29.

Young CP, Nagaswawi S. Cardiac syncope secondary to glossopharyngeal neuralgia effectively treated with carbamazepine. J Clin Psychiatry 1978;39:776–8.

Young PA, Young JA. Basic clinical neuroanatomy. Philadelphia: Williams & Wilkins; 1997. p. 292, 296.

Zigmond MJ, Bloom FE, Landis SC, et al. Fundamental neuroscience. Toronto: Academic Press; 1999. p. 1057–60, 1080–4.

X | Vagus Nerve

*carries
visceral sensation
from the larynx,
pharynx, and thoracic
and abdominal
viscera and sends
motor signals to
pharyngeal, laryngeal,
and visceral muscles*

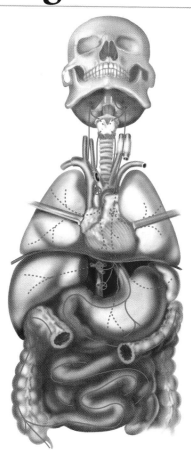

X Vagus Nerve

CASE HISTORY

Ruth is a 46-year-old lawyer who, over the last few years, noticed a whooshing sound in her left ear when she lay on her left side at night. Ruth is a very busy woman with two teenage daughters and an active law practice, and, as the noise did not keep her from sleeping at night, she paid little attention to it.

One afternoon, after playing a vigorous game of tennis with her daughter, she again became aware of the whooshing sensation in her left ear and noted that it seemed more intense with exercise. She had intended to see her family doctor but got distracted with an important defense and her daughter's upcoming graduation.

Over several months, Ruth noticed the whooshing sound was almost always present day or night, and she gradually developed problems with swallowing and a hoarse voice. Finally, Ruth made time to see her doctor.

On general examination, Ruth's doctor noted that she appeared fit and well. However, when the doctor placed a stethoscope on the base of her skull on the left side, he could hear a bruit (a whooshing sound). When he examined her cranial nerves, he found that she had an absent gag reflex on the left side and some weakness of her left sternomastoid* muscle. Ruth's doctor immediately referred her to a neurosurgeon who was concerned that this was a glomus tumor of the jugular foramen. He sent Ruth for magnetic resonance imaging (MRI) and an angiogram. The investigations confirmed the neurosurgeon's suspicions and a diagnosis of a glomus jugulare tumor was made. Ruth was subsequently scheduled for surgery to have the tumor removed.

ANATOMY OF THE VAGUS NERVE

Vagus comes from the Latin word meaning "wandering." The vagus nerve "wanders" from the brain stem to the splenic flexure of the colon. Not only is the vagus the parasympathetic nerve to the thoracic and abdominal viscera, it is also the largest visceral sensory (afferent) nerve. Sensory fibers outnumber parasympathetic fibers four to one. In the medulla, the vagal fibers are connected to four nuclei: the spinal nucleus of the trigeminal nerve (general sensory); the nucleus of the tractus solitarius (visceral sensory); the nucleus ambiguus (branchial motor); and the dorsal vagal motor nucleus (parasympathetic visceral motor) (Figure X–1 and Table X–1).

---

*Sternomastoid is a shortened form of sternocleidomastoid and will be used in this text.

Course of the Vagus Nerve

The vagus nerve emerges from the medulla of the brain stem dorsal to the olive as eight to ten rootlets caudal to those of cranial nerve IX. These rootlets converge into a flat cord that exits the skull through the jugular foramen. Two sensory ganglia, the superior (jugular) and inferior (nodosum), are located on the vagus nerve. The superior ganglion is located within the jugular fossa of the petrous temporal bone, which, together with the occipital bone, forms the jugular foramen. Within the jugular foramen, the vagus nerve is in close proximity to the jugular bulb, a swelling of the proximal part of the internal jugular vein containing the jugular glomus within its adventitia (see Case History Guiding Questions, #1). The glomus jugulare, or tympanic body, is a collection of neuron-like cells that monitor blood oxygen (O_2), carbon dioxide (CO_2), and acidity/alkalinity (pH) levels. It is similar to the carotid body (see Chapter IX). Exiting the jugular foramen, the vagus nerve enlarges into a second swelling, the inferior (nodosum) ganglion (see Figure X–1).

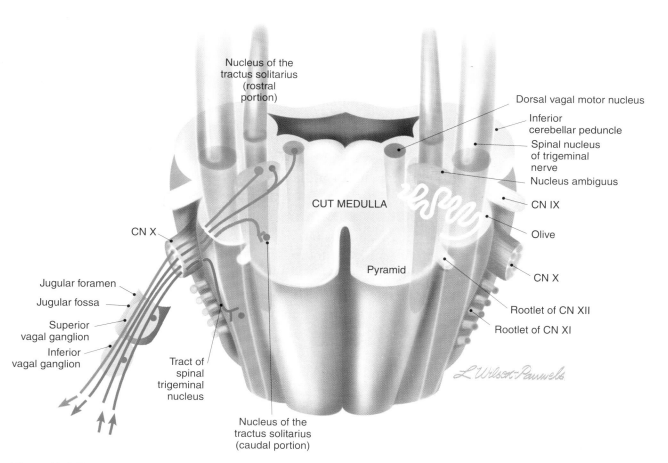

Figure X–1 Cross-section of the medulla at the point of entry of cranial nerve X illustrating the nuclei associated with this nerve.

Table X–1 Nerve Fiber Modality and Function of the Vagus Nerve

Nerve Fiber Modality*	Nucleus	Function
General sensory (afferent)	Of the spinal trigeminal tract	From the posterior meninges, concha, skin at the back of the ear and in the external acoustic meatus, part of the external surface of the tympanic membrane, the pharynx, and larnyx
Visceral sensory (afferent)	Of the tractus solitarius	From the larynx, trachea (caudal part), esophagus, and thoracic and abdominal viscera, stretch receptors in the walls of the aortic arch, and chemoreceptors in the aortic bodies adjacent to the arch
Branchial motor (efferent)	Ambiguus	To the superior, middle, and inferior constrictors, levator palati, salpingopharyngeus, palatopharyngeus, and one muscle of the tongue, the palatoglossus, via the pharyngeal plexus and to cricothyroid and intrinsic muscles of the larynx
Visceral motor (parasympathetic efferent)	Dorsal vagal motor	To smooth muscle and glands of the pharynx, larynx, and thoracic and abdominal viscera
	Ambiguus	To cardiac muscle

*Some texts list special sense for taste as one of the components of this nerve. Because cranial nerve X carries so few taste fibers, this modality has been omitted.

As the vagus nerve emerges through the jugular foramen, it lies within the same dural sheath as the accessory nerve (cranial nerve XI). For a short distance, the caudal branchial motor fibers of cranial nerve X travel with cranial nerve XI (some texts call these fibers the cranial root of XI). Just beyond the inferior ganglion, all the branchial motor fibers of cranial nerve X rejoin (Figure X–2).

In the neck, the vagus lies posterior to and in a groove between the internal jugular vein and the internal carotid artery. It descends vertically within the carotid sheath (Figure X–3), giving off branches to the pharynx, larynx, and constrictor muscles (Table X–2). The right recurrent laryngeal nerve branches from the right vagus nerve in the neck. It curves below and behind the right subclavian artery to ascend at the side of the trachea behind the right common carotid artery. The left recurrent laryngeal nerve branches from the left vagus nerve in the thorax (Figure X–4). It curves below and behind the aortic arch to ascend at the left side of the trachea. From the root of the neck downward, the vagus nerve takes a different path on each side of the body to reach the cardiac, pulmonary, and esophageal plexuses (consisting of both sympathetic and cranial nerve X parasympathetic axons). From the esophageal plexus, right and left gastric nerves arise to supply the abdominal viscera as far caudal as the splenic (left colic) flexure (see Table X–2 and Figure X–4).

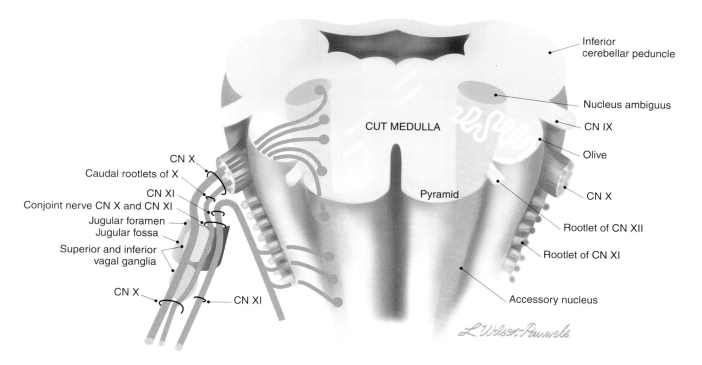

Figure X–2 Cross-section through the rostral (open) medulla demonstrating the branchial motor component of cranial nerve X including spinal rootlets of cranial nerve XI.

GENERAL SENSORY (AFFERENT) COMPONENT

The general sensory component of cranial nerve X carries sensation (pain, touch, and temperature) from the

- larynx,
- pharynx,
- concha and skin of the external ear and external auditory canal,
- external surface of the tympanic membrane, and
- meninges of the posterior cranial fossa.

Axons carrying general sensation from the vocal folds and the subglottis below the vocal folds accompany visceral sensory axons in the recurrent laryngeal nerve (Figures X–5 and X–6). Similarly, axons carrying general sensation from the larynx above the vocal folds accompany visceral sensory axons in the internal laryngeal nerve. The internal laryngeal nerve leaves the pharynx by piercing the thyrohyoid membrane. It ascends in the neck uniting with the external laryngeal nerve (branchial motor) to form the superior laryngeal nerve. General sensory fibers travel up the superior laryngeal nerve to join the rest of the vagus nerve and reach the inferior vagal ganglion.

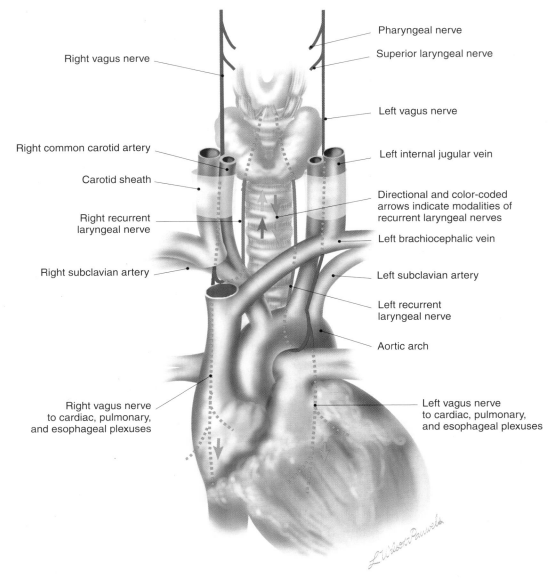

Right vagus nerve

Right common carotid artery

Carotid sheath

Right recurrent
laryngeal nerve

Right subclavian artery

Right vagus nerve
to cardiac, pulmonary,
and esophageal plexuses

Pharyngeal nerve

Superior laryngeal nerve

Left vagus nerve

Left internal jugular vein

Directional and color-coded
arrows indicate modalities of
recurrent laryngeal nerves

Left brachiocephalic vein

Left subclavian artery

Left recurrent
laryngeal nerve

Aortic arch

Left vagus nerve
to cardiac, pulmonary,
and esophageal plexuses

Figure X–3 Route of the right and left recurrent laryngeal nerves (nerve is shown in grey for clarity).

General sensory fibers from the concha and the skin of the external ear, the external auditory canal, and the external surface of the tympanic membrane are carried in the auricular branch (see Figure X–6). Stimulation of the auricular nerve of cranial nerve X in the external auditory meatus can cause reflex coughing, vomiting, and even fainting through reflex activation of the dorsal vagal motor nucleus. Sensory branches from the meninges of the posterior cranial fossa are carried in the meningeal nerve. The peripheral processes pass into the jugular fossa and enter the superior vagal ganglion where their nerve cell bodies are located.

The central processes pass upward through the jugular foramen and enter the medulla, then descend in the spinal trigeminal tract to synapse in its nucleus.

Table X–2 Branches of the Vagus Nerve

Location	Branch	General Sensory	Visceral Sensory	Branchial Motor	Visceral Motor
Jugular fossa	Meningeal	✔			
	Auricular	✔			
Neck	Pharyngeal	✔	✔	✔	✔
	Branches to carotid body		✔		
	Superior laryngeal	✔	✔	✔	✔
	Internal laryngeal	✔	✔		✔
	External laryngeal			✔	
	Recurrent laryngeal (right)	✔	✔	✔	✔
	Cardiac		✔		✔
Thorax	Cardiac		✔		✔
	Recurrent laryngeal (left)	✔	✔	✔	✔
	Pulmonary		✔		✔
	Esophageal		✔		✔
Abdomen	Gastrointestinal		✔		✔

From the nucleus of the spinal tract, second-order axons project via the ventral trigeminothalamic tract to the contralateral ventral posterior nucleus of the thalamus. Thalamic neurons project through the internal capsule to the sensory cortex of the cerebrum (see Figure X–6, inset).

VISCERAL SENSORY (AFFERENT) COMPONENT

Visceral sensation is carried in the visceral sensory component of the vagus nerve. It is not appreciated at a conscious level of awareness other than as "feeling good" or "feeling bad," unlike visceral pain that is carried in the sympathetic nervous system.

Visceral sensory fibers from plexuses around the abdominal viscera converge and join with the right and left gastric nerves of the vagus (Figure X–7). These nerves pass upward through the esophageal hiatus (opening) of the diaphragm to merge with the plexus of nerves around the esophagus. Sensory fibers from plexuses around the heart and lungs also converge with the esophageal plexus and continue up through the thorax in the right and left vagus nerves.

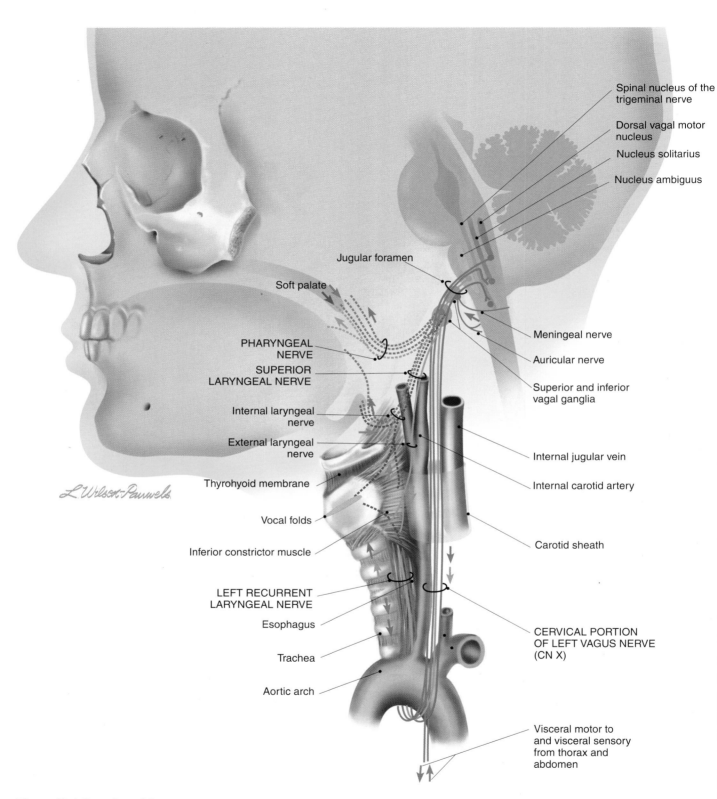

Spinal nucleus of the trigeminal nerve

Dorsal vagal motor nucleus

Nucleus solitarius

Nucleus ambiguus

Jugular foramen

Soft palate

PHARYNGEAL NERVE

SUPERIOR LARYNGEAL NERVE

Internal laryngeal nerve

External laryngeal nerve

Thyrohyoid membrane

Vocal folds

Inferior constrictor muscle

LEFT RECURRENT LARYNGEAL NERVE

Esophagus

Trachea

Aortic arch

Meningeal nerve

Auricular nerve

Superior and inferior vagal ganglia

Internal jugular vein

Internal carotid artery

Carotid sheath

CERVICAL PORTION OF LEFT VAGUS NERVE (CN X)

Visceral motor to and visceral sensory from thorax and abdomen

L. Wilson-Pauwels

Figure X–4 Overview of the vagus nerve.

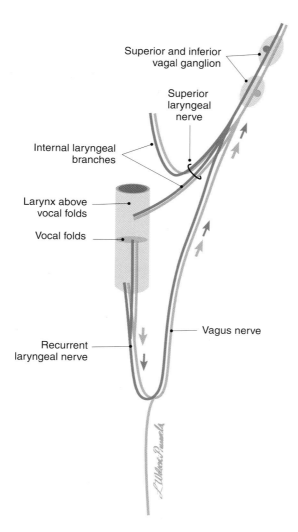

Internal laryngeal
branches

Superior and inferior
vagal ganglion

Superior
laryngeal
nerve

Larynx above
vocal folds

Vocal folds

Vagus nerve

Recurrent
laryngeal nerve

Figure X–5 Schematic illustration depicting visceral and general sensory nerves from the larynx.

The right and left vagus nerves are joined by nerves carrying visceral sensory information from the

- baroreceptors (stretch receptors) in the aortic arch and chemoreceptors (measuring oxygen tension in the blood) in the aortic bodies;
- larynx below the vocal cords in the recurrent laryngeal nerve;
- larynx above the vocal folds in the internal laryngeal nerve; and
- mucous membrane of the epiglottis, base of the tongue, and aryepiglottic folds in the pharyngeal plexus.

The central processes of the nerve cell bodies in the inferior vagal ganglion enter the medulla and descend in the tractus solitarius to enter the caudal part of the nucleus of the tractus solitarius. From the nucleus, bilateral connections important in the reflex control of cardiovascular, respiratory, and gastrointestinal functions are made with several areas of the reticular formation and the hypothalamus.

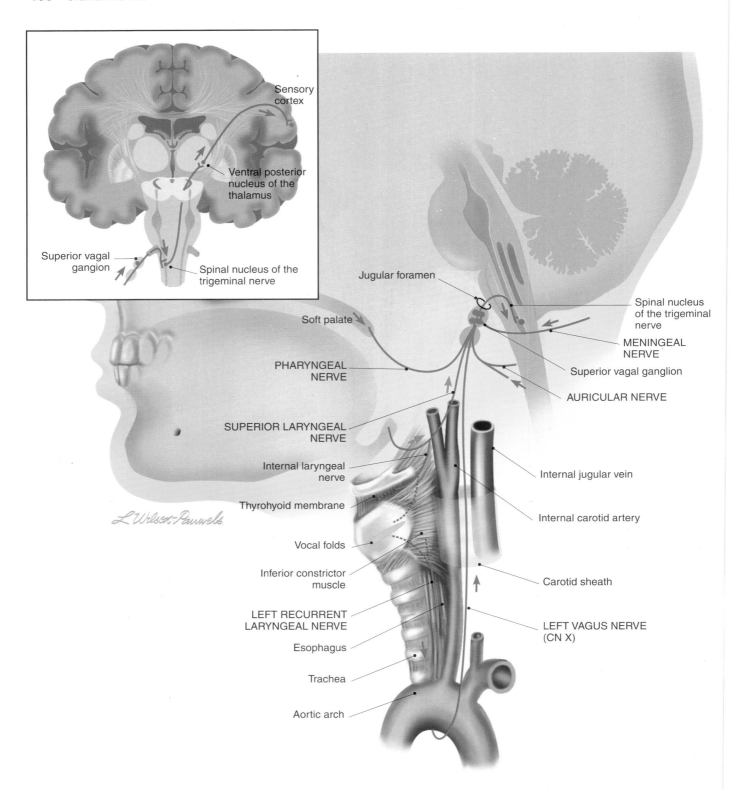

Sensory cortex

Ventral posterior nucleus of the thalamus

Superior vagal ganglion

Spinal nucleus of the trigeminal nerve

Jugular foramen

Spinal nucleus of the trigeminal nerve

MENINGEAL NERVE

Superior vagal ganglion

AURICULAR NERVE

Soft palate

PHARYNGEAL NERVE

SUPERIOR LARYNGEAL NERVE

Internal laryngeal nerve

Thyrohyoid membrane

Vocal folds

Inferior constrictor muscle

LEFT RECURRENT LARYNGEAL NERVE

Esophagus

Trachea

Aortic arch

Internal jugular vein

Internal carotid artery

Carotid sheath

LEFT VAGUS NERVE (CN X)

L. Wilson-Pauwels

Figure X–6 General sensory component of the vagus nerve.

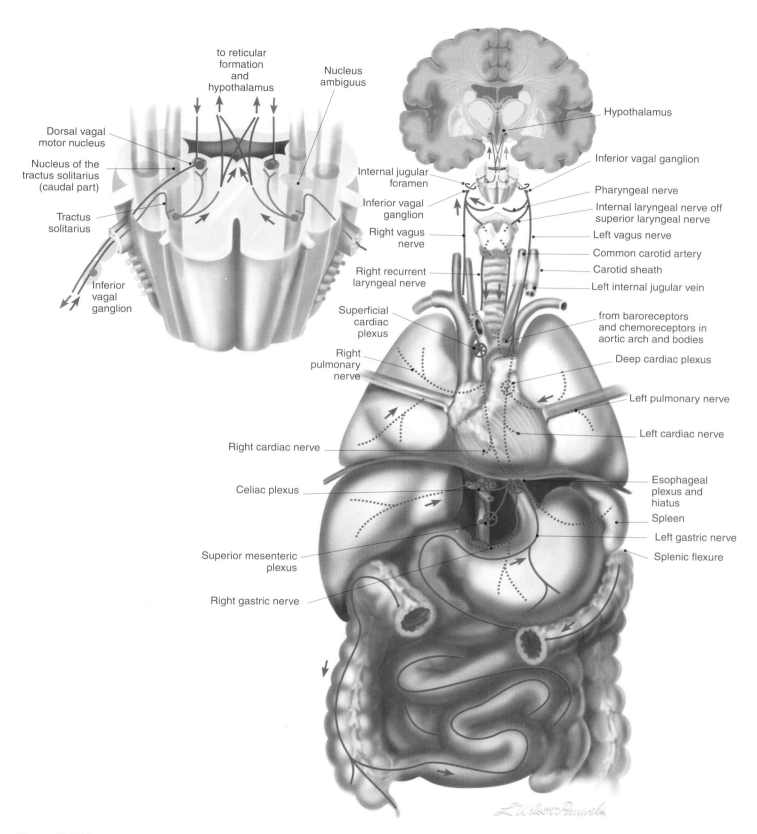

to reticular
formation
and
hypothalamus

Nucleus
ambiguus

Dorsal vagal
motor nucleus

Nucleus of the
tractus solitarius
(caudal part)

Tractus
solitarius

Inferior
vagal
ganglion

Hypothalamus

Inferior vagal ganglion

Internal jugular
foramen

Inferior vagal
ganglion

Right vagus
nerve

Right recurrent
laryngeal nerve

Pharyngeal nerve

Internal laryngeal nerve off
superior laryngeal nerve

Left vagus nerve

Common carotid artery

Carotid sheath

Left internal jugular vein

Superficial
cardiac
plexus

Right
pulmonary
nerve

from baroreceptors
and chemoreceptors in
aortic arch and bodies

Deep cardiac plexus

Left pulmonary nerve

Left cardiac nerve

Right cardiac nerve

Celiac plexus

Esophageal
plexus and
hiatus

Spleen

Left gastric nerve

Splenic flexure

Superior mesenteric
plexus

Right gastric nerve

Figure X–7 Visceral sensory component of the vagus nerve.

Connections via the reticulobulbar pathway (between the reticular formation and cranial nerve nuclei in the brain stem) to the dorsal vagal motor nucleus enable the parasympathetic fibers of the vagus nerve to control these reflex responses (see Figure X–7, inset).

BRANCHIAL MOTOR (EFFERENT) COMPONENT

Bilateral corticobulbar fibers (fibers connecting the cortex with cranial nerve nuclei in the brain stem) are composed of axons from the premotor, motor, and other cortical areas. They descend through the internal capsule to synapse on motor neurons in the nucleus ambiguus, a column of cells just dorsal to the inferior olivary nucleus in the medulla. The nucleus ambiguus also receives sensory signals from other brain stem nuclei, mainly the spinal trigeminal and solitary nuclei, initiating reflex responses (eg, coughing and vomiting). Lower motor neuron axons leave the nucleus ambiguus and travel laterally to leave the medulla as eight to ten rootlets. The caudal rootlets travel briefly with cranial nerve XI, rejoining with the rostral rootlets of cranial nerve X just below the inferior vagal ganglion (see Figure X–2). The nerve leaves the skull through the jugular foramen to reach the constrictor muscles of the pharynx and the intrinsic muscles of the larynx (see Figures X–4 and X–8).

The branchial motor fibers leave the vagus nerve as three major branches: pharyngeal, superior laryngeal, and recurrent laryngeal. The pharyngeal branch, the principal motor nerve of the pharynx, traverses the inferior ganglion and passes inferomedially between the internal and external carotid arteries. It enters the pharynx at the upper border of the middle constrictor and breaks up into the pharyngeal plexus to supply all the muscles of the pharynx and soft palate except the stylopharyngeus (cranial nerve IX) and tensor (veli) palati (branchial motor component of V_3). Therefore, it supplies the superior, middle, and inferior constrictors, levator palati, salpingopharyngeus, palatopharyngeus, and one muscle of the tongue, the palatoglossus (many are illustrated in Figure X–8).

The superior laryngeal nerve branches from the main trunk of the vagus nerve at the inferior vagal ganglion distal to the pharyngeal branch. It descends adjacent to the pharynx, dividing into internal (mainly sensory) and external (motor) laryngeal nerves. Branchial motor axons in the external laryngeal branch supply the inferior constrictor and the cricothyroid muscles. It also sends branches to the pharyngeal plexus. The pharyngeal plexus, supplying the palate and pharynx, is formed by branches from the external laryngeal and pharyngeal nerves, as well as branches from cranial nerve IX and the sympathetic trunk

The recurrent laryngeal nerve, the third major branch, takes a different path on the right and left sides of the body (see Figure X–3). The right recurrent laryngeal nerve arises from the vagus nerve anterior to the subclavian artery, then hooks back under the artery and ascends posterior to it in the groove between the trachea and the esophagus. The left recurrent laryngeal nerve arises from the left vagus on the aortic arch. It hooks back posteriorly under the arch and ascends through the

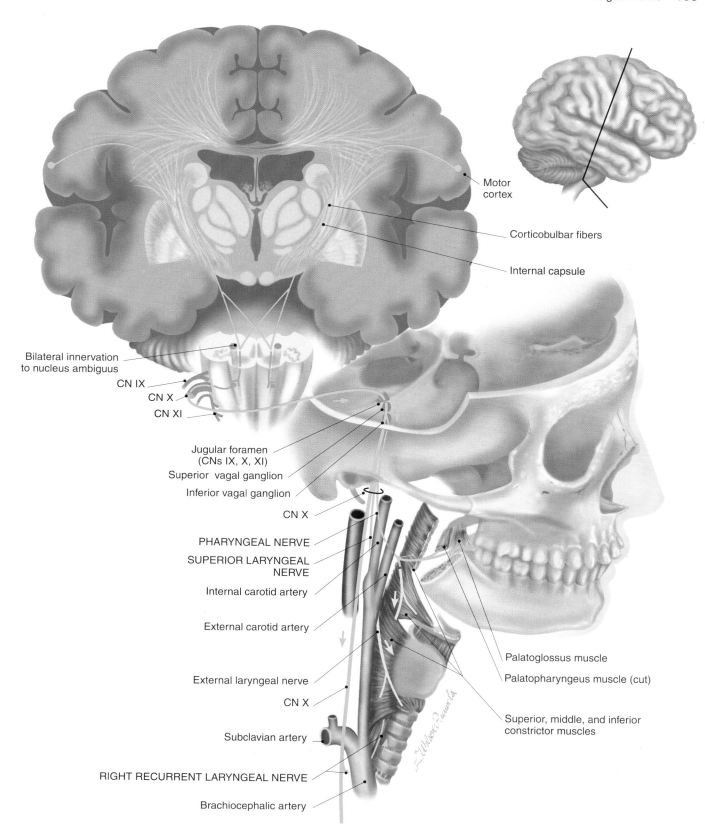

Motor cortex

Corticobulbar fibers

Internal capsule

Bilateral innervation to nucleus ambiguus

CN IX

CN X

CN XI

Jugular foramen (CNs IX, X, XI)

Superior vagal ganglion

Inferior vagal ganglion

CN X

PHARYNGEAL NERVE

SUPERIOR LARYNGEAL NERVE

Internal carotid artery

External carotid artery

External laryngeal nerve

CN X

Subclavian artery

RIGHT RECURRENT LARYNGEAL NERVE

Brachiocephalic artery

Palatoglossus muscle

Palatopharyngeus muscle (cut)

Superior, middle, and inferior constrictor muscles

Figure X–8 Branchial motor component of the vagus nerve.

superior mediastinum to reach the groove between the trachea and the esophagus on the left side. The recurrent nerves pass deep to the inferior margin of the inferior constrictor muscles. The branchial motor axons supply the intrinsic muscles of the larynx (except the cricothyroid).

VISCERAL MOTOR (PARASYMPATHETIC EFFERENT) COMPONENT

The parasympathetic nerve cell bodies of the vagus nerve are located in the dorsal motor nucleus of the vagus (Figure X–9) and in the medial side of the nucleus ambiguus. Neurons in the dorsal vagal nucleus innervate ganglia in the gut and its derivatives (lungs, liver, pancreas), whereas neurons in the nucleus ambiguus innervate ganglia in the cardiac plexus. They are all influenced by input from the hypothalamus, the olfactory system, the reticular formation, and the nucleus of the tractus solitarius. The dorsal motor nucleus of the vagus is located in the floor of the fourth ventricle (vagal trigone) and in the central gray matter of the closed medulla. Preganglionic fibers from this nucleus traverse the spinal trigeminal tract and nucleus, emerge from the lateral surface of the medulla, and travel in the vagus nerve (see Figure X–1).

Within the pharynx and larynx, the vagal preganglionic axons activate ganglionic neurons that are secretomotor to the glands of the pharyngeal and laryngeal mucosa. Preganglionic axons are distributed to the pharyngeal plexus through the pharyngeal and internal laryngeal branches (see Figure X–4). Within the thorax, the vagi take different paths, but both break up into many branches that join plexuses around the major blood vessels to the lungs and the heart (Figure X–10). Pulmonary branches cause bronchoconstriction, and esophageal branches act to speed up peristalsis in the esophagus by activating the smooth (nonstriated) muscle of the walls of the esophagus. The axons synapse in ganglia located in the walls of the individual organs. The cell bodies of cardiac preganglionic axons are located in the medial nucleus ambiguus. Their axons terminate on small ganglia associated with the heart and act to slow down the cardiac cycle.

The right and left gastric nerves emerge from the esophageal plexus. These nerves stimulate secretion by the gastric glands and are motor to the smooth muscle of the stomach. Intestinal branches act similarly on the small intestine, cecum, vermiform appendix, ascending colon, and most of the transverse colon. In the gut, the synapses occur in ganglia of the myenteric and submucosal plexuses of Auerbach and Meissner, respectively.

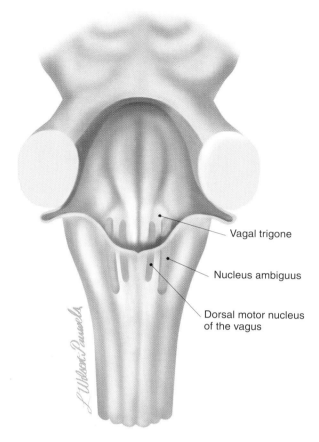

Figure X–9 Dorsal motor nucleus of the vagus nerve (posterior brain stem).

CASE HISTORY GUIDING QUESTIONS

1. What is a glomus jugulare tumor?

2. Why did Ruth hear a whooshing sound in her left ear?

3. Why did Ruth lose the gag reflex on her left side?

4. Why did Ruth develop a hoarse voice and have trouble swallowing?

5. Why was Ruth's left sternomastoid muscle weakened?

6. What other clinical signs are seen in association with a glomus jugulare tumor?

7. Where along the course of cranial nerve X can a lesion occur?

1. What is a glomus jugulare tumor?

A glomus jugulare tumor is a tumor of the glomus bodies of the jugular bulb, the proximal part of the internal jugular venous system (Figure X–11). The glomus bodies are paraganglia cells that are a part of the chemoreceptor system; therefore, like

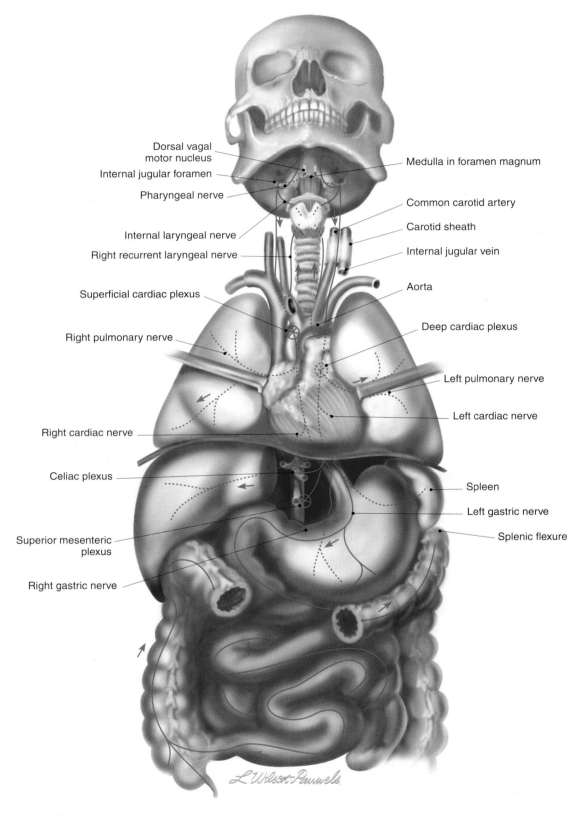

Dorsal vagal motor nucleus

Internal jugular foramen

Pharyngeal nerve

Internal laryngeal nerve

Right recurrent laryngeal nerve

Superficial cardiac plexus

Right pulmonary nerve

Right cardiac nerve

Celiac plexus

Superior mesenteric plexus

Right gastric nerve

Medulla in foramen magnum

Common carotid artery

Carotid sheath

Internal jugular vein

Aorta

Deep cardiac plexus

Left pulmonary nerve

Left cardiac nerve

Spleen

Left gastric nerve

Splenic flexure

L. Wilson-Pauwels

Figure X–10 Visceral motor component of the vagus nerve.

the carotid bodies, they monitor O_2, CO_2, and pH. The tumor typically erodes the jugular foramen resulting in compression of cranial nerves IX, X, and XI. Women are affected more often than men, and the peak incidence is during middle adult life. The treatment involves a radical mastoidectomy with removal of the tumor, followed by radiation.

2. Why did Ruth hear a whooshing sound in her left ear?

This tumor is highly vascular and, therefore, has a robust blood flow. Because it is located immediately below the floor of the middle ear, sound from the turbulent blood flow passes through the bone and stimulates the cochlea, creating a perceived whooshing noise.

3. Why did Ruth lose the gag reflex on her left side?

The gag reflex involves the sensory afferents from cranial nerve IX and the motor efferents of cranial nerve X (Figures X–12 and X–13). If either limb of the reflex arc is damaged, the gag reflex will be lost. In Ruth's case, the tumor compromised both the sensory (cranial nerve IX) and the motor limbs (cranial nerve X) of the gag reflex.

4. Why did Ruth develop a hoarse voice and have trouble swallowing?

When the muscles controlling one of the vocal cords are paralysed by loss of their innervation, the cord becomes lax and cannot vibrate against the other cord. As a result, the voice becomes low pitched and hoarse. The patient, having to force increased amounts of air to set the intact cord in motion, becomes short of breath when speaking. Also, the impairment causes difficulty swallowing due to an inability to elevate the soft palate adequately (unilateral loss of levator palati muscle). This may allow food to pass up the nose.

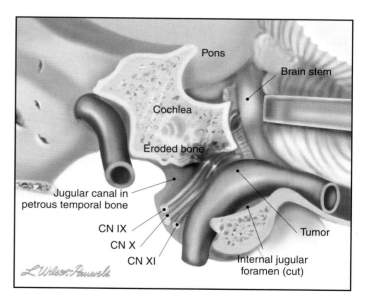

Figure X–11 Tumor of the glomus bodies of the jugular bulb compressing cranial nerves IX, X, and XI (lateral view showing cut internal jugular foramen).

5. Why was Ruth's left sternomastoid muscle weakened?

The sternomastoid muscle is innervated by the accessory nerve (cranial nerve XI) that exits the skull through the jugular foramen. The tumor has compressed and compromised the accessory nerve (see Figure X–11).

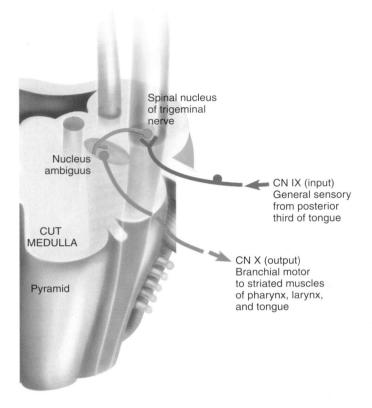

Figure X–12 Gag reflex involving cranial nerve IX (input) and cranial nerve X (output).

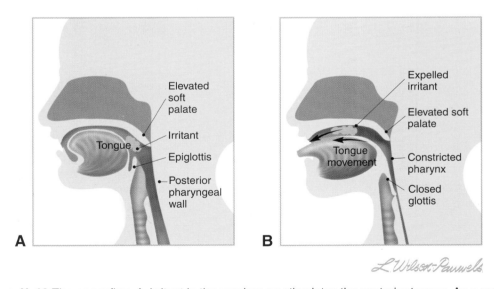

Figure X–13 The gag reflex. *A*, Irritant in the oropharynx stimulates the posterior tongue. As a result, cranial nerve IX's general sensory afferent nerve fibers are stimulated. *B*, A reflex response by cranial nerve X cell bodies in the nucleus ambiguus stimulates branchial motor efferent nerves resulting in elevation of the soft palate, closure of the glottis, and contraction of the pharyngeal wall to expel the foreign object.

6. What other clinical signs are seen in association with a glomus jugulare tumor?

The glomus jugulare tumor is an invasive tumor that has multiple extensions and will spread into any hole or fissure in the petrous temporal bone. Clinical signs are the result of invasion of the tumor and compression of adjacent nerves. The typical syndrome consists of a systolic bruit (abnormal sound or murmur), partial deafness, dysphagia (difficulty in swallowing), and dysphonia (difficulty in speaking) because of damage to cranial nerves VIII, IX, and X.

Other neurologic findings are correlated with the extension of the tumor. If the tumor

* spreads toward the foramen magnum, there may be a cranial nerve XII palsy (paresis or paralysis of tongue muscles);
* invades the intrapetrous carotid canal, a Horner's syndrome, characterized by miosis (constricted pupil), ptosis (drooping of the eyelid), enophthalmos (recession of the eyeball), and redness and dry skin on the ipsilateral face, may develop due to sympathetic nerve involvement;
* spreads into the inner ear, there may be vestibular (balance) and cochlear (diminished hearing) involvement; or
* extends directly into the external auditory canal, a vascular tumor may be visualized.

7. Where along the course of cranial nerve X can a lesion occur?

A lesion of the vagus nerve can occur anywhere along its course from the cortex to the organ of innervation. An upper motor neuron lesion (UMNL) can occur anywhere between the cortex and the nucleus ambiguus. Lesions that involve these fibers are typically ischemias (insufficient blood supply), infarcts, or tumors. Bilateral UMNLs involving the corticobulbar tracts affect the bulbar* musculature and are referred to as a pseudobulbar palsy. This is a misleading term as there is nothing "pseudo" about a palsy. Spastic bulbar palsy would be a better term.

A lesion at the level of the nucleus ambiguus and below is a lower motor neuron lesion (LMNL). A unilateral lesion of the lower motor neuron fibers results in a bulbar palsy (light or incomplete paralysis) of the bulbar muscles on the ipsilateral side. Lower motor neuron lesions can occur from mass lesions compressing the pons, from tumors of the jugular foramen, and from surgical mishaps following procedures in the neck area such as a carotid endarterectomy or a thyroidectomy. The LMNLs also can occur from compression of the left recurrent laryngeal nerve by lung tumors or paratracheal lymph nodes compressing the nerve as it passes through the thorax.

---

*The term bulbar means a swelling. In neurology, we use the term bulbar to refer to the medulla and/or brain stem. Since corticobulbar tracts are those that go from the cortex to the brain stem to synapse on nuclei there, they are named corticobulbar. Muscles supplied by these nerves are called "bulbar" muscles.

CLINICAL TESTING

Cranial nerve X is usually tested in conjuction with cranial nerve IX by assessment of the gag reflex. However, it is possible to test cranial nerve X in isolation. A unilateral lesion of the nerve results in lowering and flattening of the palatal arch on the affected side. Therefore, when examining the tenth nerve, one should observe the posterior pharynx at rest and then on phonation. On phonation, there is contraction of the superior pharyngeal muscle. Unilateral paresis of the superior pharyngeal constrictor results in deviation of the uvula to the normal side and also a pull of the posterior pharyngeal wall toward the intact side (Figure X–14). Because the damaged side cannot counter the pull of the intact side, the motion resembles that of swagging or drawing a curtain (of pharyngeal muscles) to the unaffected side, as you would swag a drape to the side. (See also Cranial Nerves Examination on CD-ROM.)

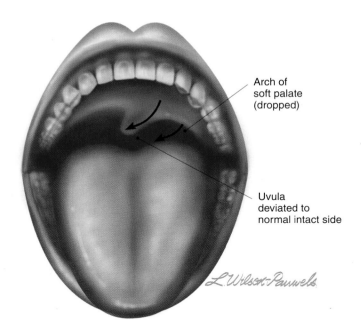

Arch of
soft palate
(dropped)

Uvula
deviated to
normal intact side

Figure X–14 Lower motor neuron lesion (LMNL) on the left side.

ADDITIONAL RESOURCES

Bradley WG, Daroff RB, Fenichel GM, Marsden CD. Neurology in clinical practice. 2nd ed. Toronto: Butterworth-Heinemann; 1996. p. 251–63.

Brodal A. Neurological anatomy in relation to clinical medicine. 3rd ed. New York, Oxford: Oxford University Press; 1981. p. 460, 464, 712.

Fitzerald MTJ. Neuroanatomy basic and clinical. 3rd ed. Toronto: W.B. Saunders Company Ltd; 1996. p. 148–50.

George B. Jugulare paragangliomas. Acta Neurochir (Wien) 1992;118:20–6.

Kandel ER, Schwartz JH, Jessell TM. Principles of neuroscience. 3rd ed. New York: Elsevier; 1991. p. 772.

Kiernan JA. Barr's the human nervous system. 7th ed. Phildelphia, New York: Lippincott-Raven; 1998. p. 169–74.

Kramer W. Glomus jugulare tumors. Handbook of clinical neurology. Vol 18. Amsterdam, Holland: Baillière and Tindall; 1975. p. 435–55.

Lindsay WK, Bone I, Callander R. Neurology and neurosurgery illustrated. 3rd ed. New York: Churchill Livingstone; 1997. p. 172–3, 343.

Nolte J. The human brain. 4th ed. Toronto: Mosby; 1999. p. 291, 306.

Sillars HA, Fagan PA. The management of multiple paraganglioma of the head and neck. Laryngol Otol 1993;107:538–42.

XI Accessory Nerve

*innervates the
sternomastoid
muscle and the
upper fibers
of the
trapezius
muscle*

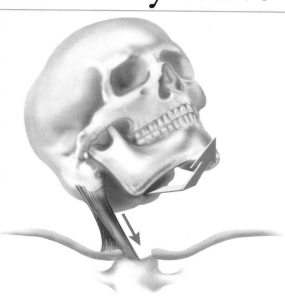

XI Accessory Nerve

CASE HISTORY

Burt, a 55-year-old businessman, was having episodes of weakness involving his right face and arm. These were diagnosed as transient ischemic attacks (TIAs) often referred to as reversible strokes. During investigation for his TIAs, he was found to have 90 percent narrowing of his left internal carotid artery and underwent left carotid endarterectomy.

Approximately two weeks postoperatively, Burt began to notice he was having problems pulling a sweater off over his head and was unable to bring his left arm over his head while swimming. He also developed a constant aching on the left side of his neck and left ear and a dull pain in his left shoulder. The vascular surgeon referred Burt to a neurologist. The neurologist noted that sensation was intact over Burt's face, neck, and shoulders, but he had weakness with shoulder elevation on his left side and was unable to abduct (raise) his left arm above the level of his shoulder. Electromyographic and nerve conduction studies showed that there had been damage to the branch of the left accessory (spinal) nerve that supplies the trapezius muscle, but that the branch to the sternomastoid* muscle had been spared.

ANATOMY OF THE ACCESSORY NERVE

Information from the premotor association cortex and other cortical areas is fed into the motor cortex by association fibers. Axons of cortical neurons descend in the corticospinal† tract through the posterior limb of the internal capsule. Cortical neurons destined to supply the sternomastoid muscle descend to the ipsilateral accessory (spinal) nucleus located in the lateral part of the anterior grey column of the upper five or six segments of the cervical spinal cord, approximately in line with the nucleus ambiguus. Axons designated to supply the trapezius muscle cross the midline in the pyramidal decussation to synapse in the contralateral accessory nucleus (Figure XI–1 and Table XI–1).

From the accessory nucleus, postsynaptic fibers emerge from the lateral white matter of the spinal cord as a series of rootlets to form the accessory nerve (see Figure XI–1 and Chapter X, Figure X–2). The rootlets emerge posterior to the ligamentum denticulatum, but anterior to the dorsal roots of the spinal cord (Figure XI–2). The rootlets form a nerve trunk that ascends rostrally in the subarachnoid space and parallel to the spinal cord as far as the foramen magnum. At the foramen magnum,

---

*Sternomastoid is a shortened form of sternocleidomastoid and will be used in this text.
†The term corticospinal tract versus corticobulbar tract is used because the descending axons project to the accessory nucleus in the spinal cord rather than to a nucleus in the brain stem.

Table XI–1 Nerve Fiber Modality and Function of the Accessory Nerve

Nerve Fiber Modality	Nucleus	Function
Branchial motor (efferent)	Accessory (spinal)	To supply sternomastoid and trapezius muscles

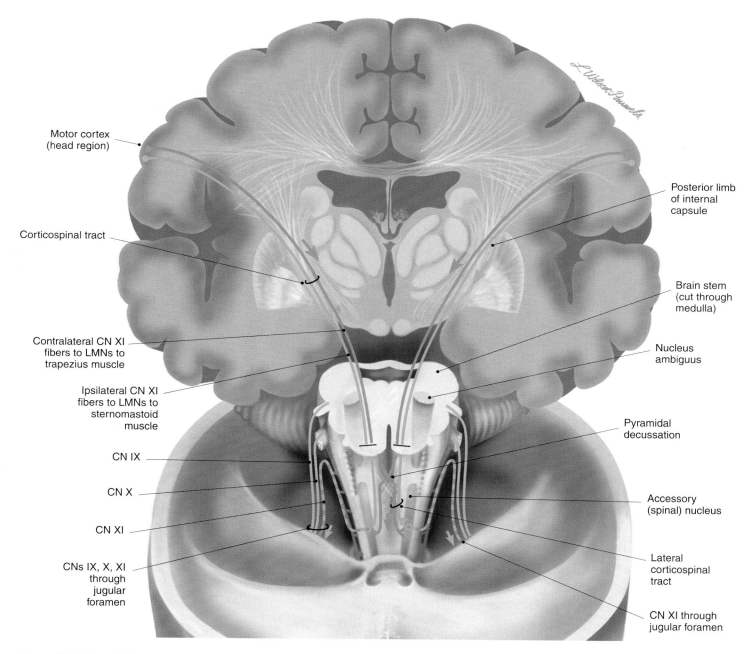

Figure XI–1 Branchial motor component of cranial nerve XI demonstrating ipsilateral innervation to LMNs innervating the sternomastoid muscle (yellow) and contralateral innervation to LMNs innervating the trapezius muscle (ochre). The brain stem is elevated. LMNs = lower motor neurons.

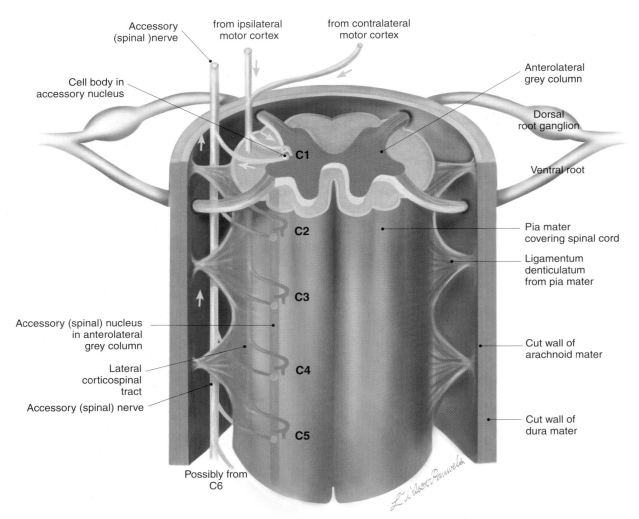

Figure XI–2 Branchial motor component of the accessory (spinal) nerve—C1 to C5 or C6.

the nerve passes posterior to the vertebral artery, to enter the posterior cranial fossa. The fibers join with caudal fibers from cranial nerve X and then separate from them within the jugular foramen (see Chapter X, Figure X–2).

As the accessory nerve emerges from the jugular foramen, it passes posteriorly, medial to the styloid process, descends obliquely, and enters the upper portion of the sternomastoid muscle on its deep surface. Some of the fibers terminate in this muscle, and the remaining fibers pass through the muscle to emerge at the midpoint of its posterior border. These fibers then cross the posterior triangle of the neck, superficial to the levator scapulae where they are closely related to the superficial cervical lymph nodes. Five centimeters above the clavicle, the nerve passes deep to the anterior border of the trapezius* to supply this muscle (Figure XI–3).

---

*There is some controversy whether branches from cervical nerves III and IV also contribute somatic motor fibers to the trapezius muscle or whether they supply only sensory fibers to the area.

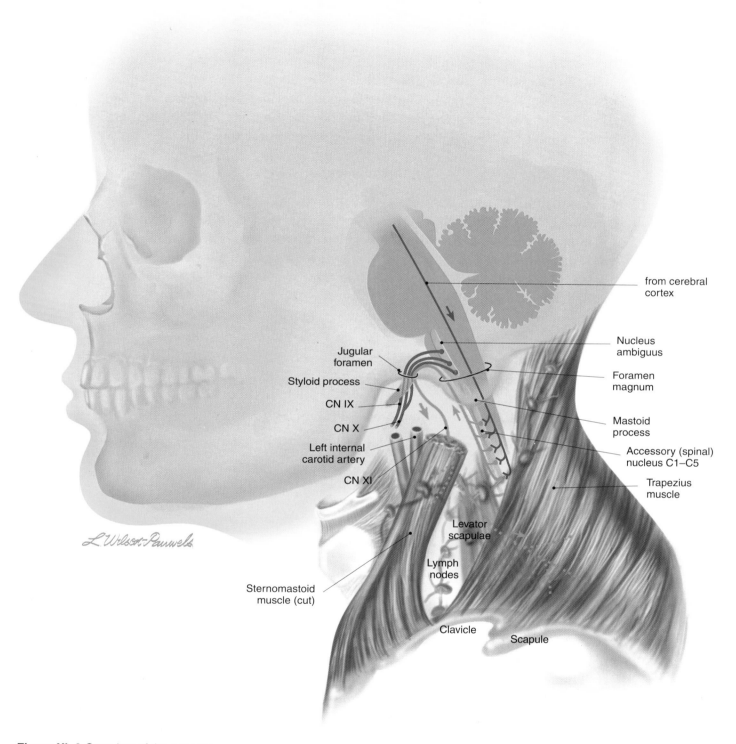

Figure XI–3 Overview of the accessory nerve.

The accessory nucleus is considered by some authors to be somatic motor to the sternomastoid and trapezius muscles. Others describe it as branchial motor to these same muscles and still others describe it as mixed somatic motor and branchial motor. In this book, the nucleus is considered to be branchial motor because it occupies a position in the ventral horn that is in line with other branchial motor nuclei. Also, its rootlets exit from the cord in the same position as other branchial motor rootlets (ie, between somatic motor and sensory rootlets).

Accessory Nerve

In this text, the accessory nerve is defined as the axons of only those lower motor neurons (LMNs) that form the accessory nucleus. Some other textbooks describe the accessory nerve as having both a rostral/cranial root (axons from the nucleus ambiguus traveling with cranial nerve X) and a caudal/spinal root (axons from the accessory nucleus, cranial nerve XI). See Chapter X and Figure X–2 for a further explanation.

CASE HISTORY GUIDING QUESTIONS

1. What is the function of the sternomastoid muscle?

2. Why are the right sternomastoid and left trapezius muscles controlled by the same side of the cortex?

3. In Burt's case, how did his cranial nerve XI get damaged? Why is his trapezius muscle affected and his sternomastoid muscle spared?

4. What else could cause an isolated accessory nerve palsy?

5. If the accessory nerve is strictly motor in function, why is Burt experiencing pain?

1. What is the function of the sternomastoid muscle?

The sternomastoid muscle acts to pull the mastoid process toward the clavicle, resulting in a rotation of the head and an elevation of the chin to the opposite side (Figure XI–4). The lower motor neurons (LMNs) that innervate the right sternomastoid muscle receive ipsilateral input from the right cortex via the accessory nerve.

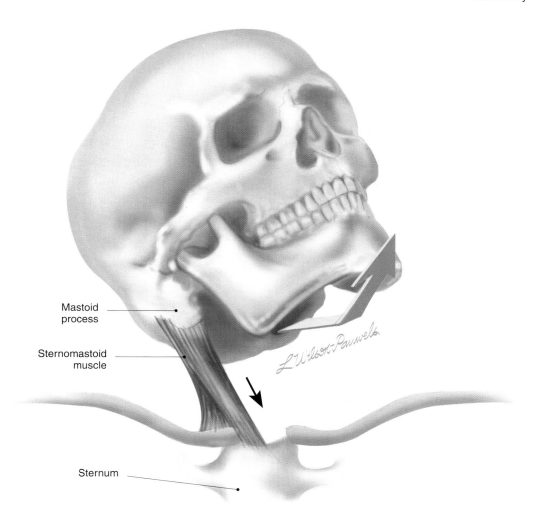

Figure XI–4 Action of the right sternomastoid muscle.

2. Why are the right sternomastoid and left trapezius muscles controlled by the same side of the cortex?

When the left upper limb muscles (including trapezius) are being used to manipulate an object, the head is turned to the left side to see what is happening. It is the right sternomastoid muscle that turns the head to the left. However, it is the left trapezius muscle that elevates the shoulder. Therefore, the right cortex controls all the muscles necessary to perform these actions.

Right cortex → Right LMNs to ipsilateral sternomastoid muscle → Chin elevates and head turns to left

Right cortex → Left LMNs to contralateral trapezius muscle → Left shoulder elevates

3. In Burt's case, how did his cranial nerve XI get damaged? Why is his trapezius muscle affected and his sternomastoid muscle spared?

The accessory nerve usually gives off branches to the sternomastoid prior to entering the muscle. The nerve then traverses the muscle and crosses the posterior triangle of the neck to reach and supply the trapezius muscle (see Figure XI–3).

During Burt's carotid endarterectomy surgery, the sternomastoid muscle was retracted to fully expose the common carotid artery. If the retraction is too vigorous, it has the potential to stretch and selectively damage the branch of the spinal accessory nerve to the trapezius lying within the sternomastoid muscle. This is what happened to Burt.

4. What else could cause an isolated accessory nerve palsy?

An isolated accessory nerve palsy is uncommon; however, the accessory nerve can be damaged during surgical procedures on the neck (eg, lymph node biopsy or internal jugular vein cannulation). In addition, trauma, including carrying heavy loads on the shoulder, attempted suicide by hanging, and neck bites sustained during passionate sex, can damage the accessory nerve. It is the axons that supply the trapezius muscle that are the most vulnerable to damage, since they take a long course through the posterior triangle of the neck (see Figure XI–3). The axons to the sternomastoid muscle, which leave the main trunk high in the neck, are relatively spared.

5. If the accessory nerve is strictly motor in function, why is Burt experiencing pain?

Burt is experiencing pain because his inactive trapezius muscle is no longer supporting his shoulder, and the remaining shoulder and arm muscles are required to assume an unaccustomed load. The resulting muscle fatigue and strain on the muscles and ligaments results in pain in his left shoulder, lateral neck, and periauricular regions. His pain can be relieved by support of the arm at the elbow with a sling.

CLINICAL TESTING

The accessory nerve is a purely motor nerve that supplies the sternomastoid and trapezius muscles. Each of these muscles should be tested separately because, as in Burt's case, it is possible to have a partial accessory nerve palsy affecting only one of these muscles.

The initial step involved in testing the accessory nerve is the assessment of the bulk of the sternomastoid and trapezius muscles. If there has been damage to the nerve (LMN lesion) there may be evidence of wasting of the muscle. Once muscle bulk is assessed then strength should be tested. (See also Cranial Nerves Examination on CD-ROM.)

Assessment of the Sternomastoid Muscle

The sternomastoid muscle functions to tilt the face and elevate the chin to the opposite side. Therefore, by asking the patient to tilt the face up and toward the opposite side, one can assess the bulk of the muscle by viewing and palpating it (Figure XI–5). The strength of this muscle is assessed by asking the patient to tilt his chin toward the opposite side against resistance.

Assessment of the Trapezius Muscle

The trapezius muscle functions to retract the head and to elevate, retract, and rotate the scapula. To assess the bulk of this muscle, it is important to expose the shoulder fully. A wasted trapezius muscle may result in a downward and lateral rotation of the scapula and some shoulder drop on the affected side. This can be seen when looking at the patient's back (Figure XI–6).

The innervation of the trapezius muscle is variably described, but it is generally agreed that the upper fibers of the trapezius are innervated by the accessory nerve.

The upper fibers of the trapezius muscle are responsible for elevation and upward rotation of the scapula enabling abduction of the arm beyond 90 degrees. To assess the strength, ask the patient to abduct the arm through 180 degrees. The examiner applies resistance to the outstretched arm once the arm is beyond 90 degrees. The trapezius can also be tested by asking the patient to shrug his shoulders against resistance (Figure XI–7). However, make sure the patient is not bracing his hands against his legs to keep the trapezius muscle elevated.

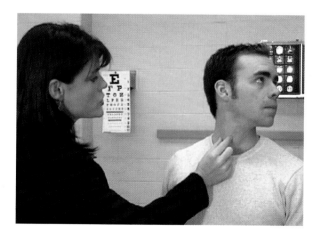

Figure XI–5 Examination and palpation of the right sternomastoid muscle.

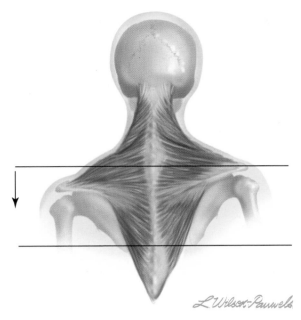

Figure XI–6 Left shoulder drop — resulting from loss of action of upper fibers of the trapezius muscle.

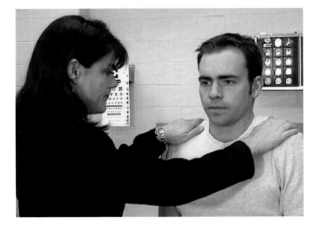

Figure XI–7 Patient shrugging his shoulders against resistance.

ADDITIONAL RESOURCES

Brodal A. Neurological anatomy in relation to clinical medicine. 3rd ed. New York: Oxford University Press; 1981. p. 457–8.

Fitzerald MTJ. Neuroanatomy basic and clinical. 3rd ed. Toronto: W.B. Saunders Company Ltd; 1996. p.144–8, 150.

Glick TH. Neurologic skills. In: Examination and diagnosis. New York: Blackwell Science Publications; 1993. p. 101.

Haines DE. Fundamental neuroscience. New York: Churchill Livingstone; 1997. p. 357.

Hoffman JC. Permanent paralysis of the accessory nerve after cannulation of the internal jugular vein. Anesthesiology 1984;58:583–4.

Kiernan JA. Barr's the human nervous system. 7th ed. Phildelphia, New York: Lippincott-Raven; 1998. p. 171–3.

Lindsay WK, Bone I, Callander R. Neurology and neurosurgery illustrated. 3rd ed. New York: Churchill Livingstone; 1997. p. 174.

Logigian EL, McInnes JM, Berger AR, et al. Stretch induced spinal accessory nerve palsy. Muscle Nerve 1988;11:146–50.

Maiglia AJ, Han DP. Cranial nerve injuries following carotid endarterectomy: an analysis of 336 procedures. Head Neck 1991;13:121–4.

Paljarvi L, Partanen J. Biting palsy of the accessory nerve. J Neurol Neurosurg Psychiatry 1980;43:744–6.

Sweeney PJ, Wilbourn AJ. Spinal accessory (11th) nerve palsy following carotid endarterectomy. Neurology 1992;42:674–5.

XII | Hypoglossal Nerve

innervates
extrinsic
and
intrinsic muscles
of the
tongue

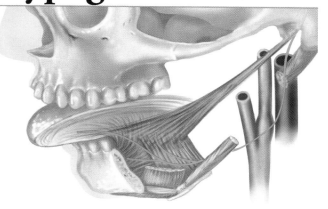

XII Hypoglossal Nerve

CASE HISTORY

Todd is a 34-year-old bodybuilder. One afternoon while lifting weights at the gym, he experienced a sudden onset of pain in the left side of his neck radiating to his head. He had no other symptoms, but the pain was sufficient to make him stop his workout. The next day the pain had almost disappeared, but over breakfast he noticed he had difficulty moving food around in his mouth, his tongue felt heavy, and his speech was slurred.

Concerned that he had experienced a stroke, Todd went to the hospital. When examined, his eye movements and pupillary reflexes were normal. All his cranial nerves functioned normally except cranial nerve XII. When he was asked to protrude his tongue it deviated to the left. He was then asked to push his tongue into his right cheek and hold it there. The doctor was able to push the tongue toward the midline. Todd's taste and general sensation of the tongue were intact. All his other motor and sensory functions were normal.

A computed tomography (CT) scan of Todd's head was normal. An angiogram was done to look at blood flow to the brain. This test showed that Todd had suffered a dissecting aneurysm of the left internal carotid artery, which narrowed the lumen, thereby restricting blood flow and in addition caused a bulging of the vessel wall outwards. However, the angiogram also demonstrated that the left cerebral hemisphere was still well perfused with blood from the collateral blood supply to the circle of Willis.

ANATOMY OF THE HYPOGLOSSAL NERVE

The rootlets of the hypoglossal nerve emerge from the anterior surface of the medulla in the ventrolateral sulcus between the pyramid and the olive. They converge to form the hypoglossal nerve, which exits the cranium through the hypoglossal (anterior condylar) foramen in the posterior cranial fossa. After exiting the skull, the nerve courses medial to cranial nerves IX, X, and XI. It passes laterally and downwards close to the posterior surface of the inferior ganglion of the vagus nerve to lie between the internal carotid artery and the internal jugular vein and deep to the posterior belly of the digastric muscle. Crossing lateral to the bifurcation of the common carotid artery, the nerve loops anteriorly above the greater cornu of the hyoid bone. It runs on the lateral surface of the hyoglossus muscle and passes deep to the intermediate tendon of the digastric muscle, the stylohyoid muscle, and the free posterior border of the mylohyoid muscle. It then passes forward on the lateral surface of the genioglossus muscle, dividing to supply its target muscles (Figure XII–1 and Table XII–1).

Table XII–1 Nerve Fiber Modality and Function of the Hypoglossal Nerve

Nerve Fiber Modality	Nucleus	Function
Somatic motor (efferent)	Hypoglossal	To supply three of the four <u>ex</u>trinsic muscles of the tongue (ie, genioglossus, styloglossus, and hyoglossus) and all <u>in</u>trinsic muscles of the tongue

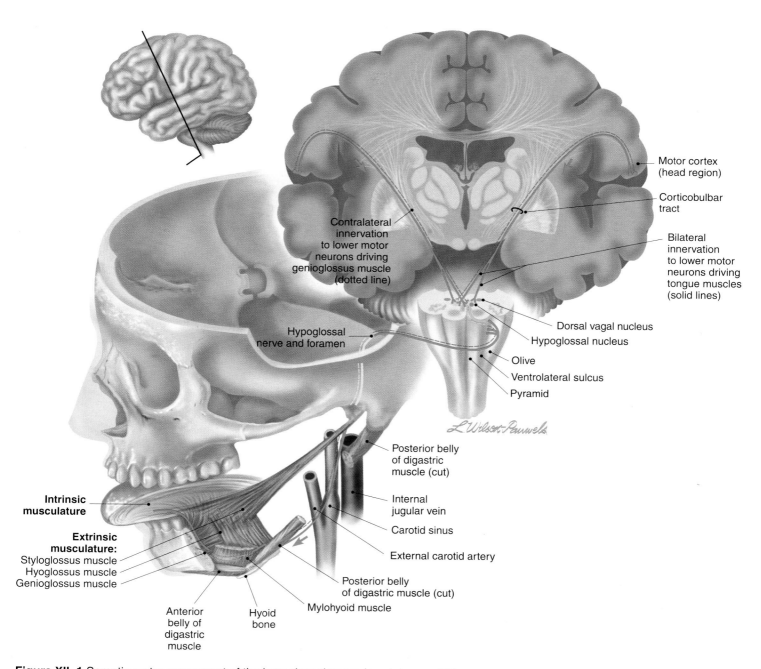

Figure XII–1 Somatic motor component of the hypoglossal nerve (cranial nerve XII).

The hypoglossal nerve supplies all the intrinsic muscles and all but one of the extrinsic muscles of the tongue, the exception being the palatoglossus muscle, which is supplied by cranial nerve X. The intrinsic muscles act to change the shape of the tongue. The extrinsic muscles act to protrude, elevate, and retract the tongue, as well as move it from side to side. The tongue has two very important functions. The phylogenetically "old" function is concerned with eating and swallowing. These actions occur in response to sensory signals from the mouth. Gustatory (taste) and tactile (touch) signals pass from the mouth through the nucleus of the tractus solitarius, the trigeminal nucleus, and the reticular formation to act on the hypoglossal nucleus resulting in reflex activities such as swallowing, sucking, and chewing. The intricate and complex movements of the tongue in speech constitute the phylogenetically "new" function of the tongue. Information from the inferior frontal cortex, premotor association cortex, and other cortical areas is projected to the primary motor area (precentral gyrus) of the cortex, which, in turn, sends signals to the hypoglossal nuclei via the corticobulbar tracts. Most of these projections are bilateral, with one exception: the cortical neurons that drive the genioglossus muscles project only to the contralateral hypoglossal nucleus.

The hypoglossal nucleus (Figure XII–2) is composed of lower motor neurons whose axons form the hypoglossal nerve. It is located in the tegmentum of the medulla between the dorsal nucleus of the vagus and the midline. It is a long thin nucleus that is approximately coextensive with the olive. It extends rostrally to form the hypoglossal triangle in the floor of the fourth ventricle (see Figure XII–2B). Axons from the hypoglossal nucleus pass ventrally to the lateral side of the medial lemniscus to emerge as a number of rootlets in the ventrolateral sulcus between the olive and the pyramid. Because the hypoglossal nuclei are located very close together, a nuclear lesion tends to affect both nuclei, causing bilateral loss of innervation to the tongue.

CASE HISTORY GUIDING QUESTIONS

1. How could Todd have damaged cranial nerve XII?

2. What other cranial nerves could be damaged by this process?

3. Why could Todd still experience sensation from his tongue?

4. How would you differentiate between an upper motor neuron lesion (UMNL) and a lower motor neuron lesion (LMNL)?

5. What findings confirmed that Todd had a lower motor neuron lesion?

6. Why were there no signs of fasciculations and atrophy of Todd's tongue?

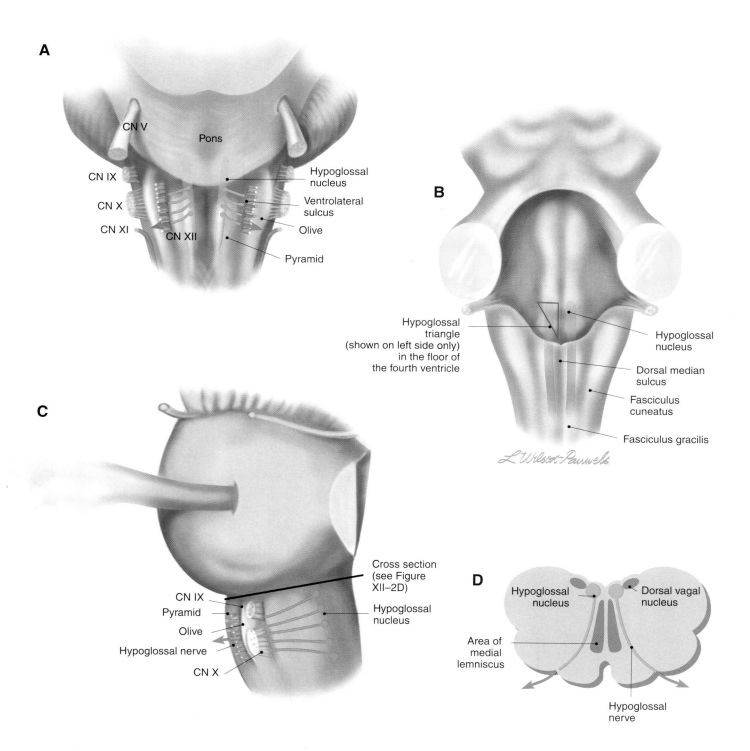

Figure XII–2 Views of the hypoglossal nucleus. *A*, Ventral view. *B*, Dorsal view. *C*, Lateral view. *D*, Cross-section through the medulla—open portion.

1. How could Todd have damaged cranial nerve XII?

While straining lifting weights, Todd tore the lining of his left internal carotid artery. Because of the tear, blood flowed between the tunica intima and tunica media of the artery wall and formed a blood clot. This splitting of the layers of the vessel wall is referred to as an arterial dissection (Figure XII–3). The blood clot narrowed the lumen of the vessel, decreasing blood flow, and significantly expanding the circumference of the internal carotid artery, thereby compressing the adjacent cranial nerve XII where it crossed the artery (Figure XII–4).

2. What cranial nerves could be damaged by this process?

Any nerves that lie in close proximity to the internal carotid artery could be affected. The most commonly affected are cranial nerves IX, X, and XII. Isolated cranial nerve palsies such as Todd's are a rare presentation associated with internal carotid artery dissection. More commonly, an internal carotid artery dissection results in occlusion of the artery. If collateral blood flow through the circle of Willis is not sufficient, the ipsilateral cerebral hemisphere is deprived of blood, leading to focal cerebral deficits.

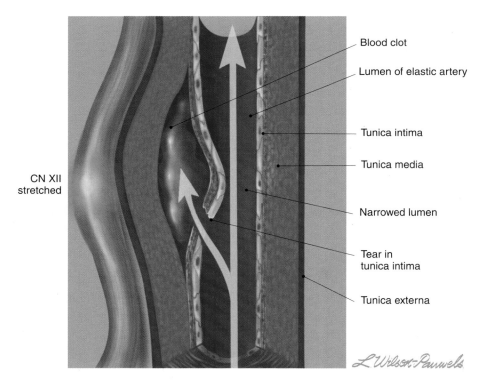

Figure XII–3 Carotid artery dissection demonstrating a blood clot between the tunica intima and the tunica media of the internal carotid artery.

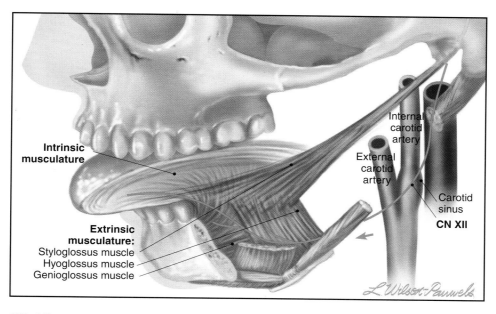

Figure XII–4 Demonstrating the hypoglossal nerve (cranial nerve XII) crossing the bifurcation of the internal and external carotid artery.

3. Why could Todd still experience sensation from his tongue?

Taste sensation from the tongue is carried primarily by cranial nerves VII and IX, while general sensation from the tongue is carried in the mandibular division of cranial nerve V and by cranial nerve IX. These modalities were spared because the nerves that carry them are not located close enough to the damaged area of the artery to be affected.

4. How would you differentiate between an upper motor neuron lesion (UMNL) and a lower motor neuron lesion (LMNL)?*

The genioglossus is one of the most clinically important extrinsic tongue muscles because, unlike the other tongue muscles, its nucleus is not bilaterally innervated. When the genioglossi muscles contract together, the tongue sticks straight out (Figure XII–5). If one genioglossus muscle can contract and the other cannot, the tongue will deviate toward the inactive side.

---

*See description of upper versus lower motor neuron lesions in the introductory chapter.

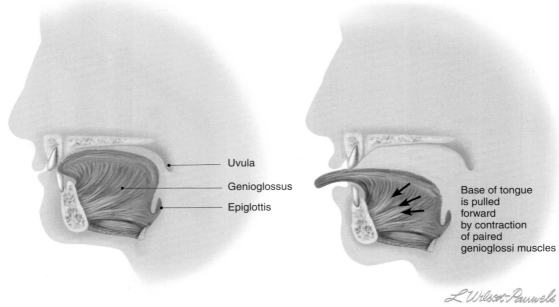

Uvula

Genioglossus

Epiglottis

Base of tongue
is pulled
forward
by contraction
of paired
genioglossi muscles

L Wilson-Pauwels

Figure XII–5 Action of the genioglossus in sticking out the tongue.

Damage to the upper motor neuron (UMNL) anywhere along the path of the axon from the cerebral cortex to the contralateral hypoglossal nucleus might result in paralysis of the contralateral genioglossus muscle. In this case, the tongue would deviate to the side opposite to the lesion (Figure XII–6).

When the lower motor neuron is damaged (LMNL) anywhere between the hypoglossal nucleus and the tongue, there is flaccid paralysis of the ipsilateral half of the tongue with fasciculation and atrophy of tongue muscles on the affected side. In this case, the ipsilateral genioglossus muscle would be paralysed and the tongue would deviate to the same side as the lesion (Figure XII–7).

5. What findings confirmed that Todd had a lower motor neuron lesion?

Two findings confirmed that Todd had a LMNL. The angiogram demonstrated that Todd had a dissection in the wall of the left internal carotid artery where it could compress the hypoglossal nerve (see Figure XII–3), and Todd's tongue deviated to the left side (see Figure XII–7).

6. Why were there no signs of fasciculations and atrophy of Todd's tongue?

When a muscle is denervated it usually takes a couple of weeks for fasciculations and atrophy to be noticeable. Todd was seen the day after his accident; therefore, fasciculations and atrophy of his left tongue muscles would not have had time to develop.

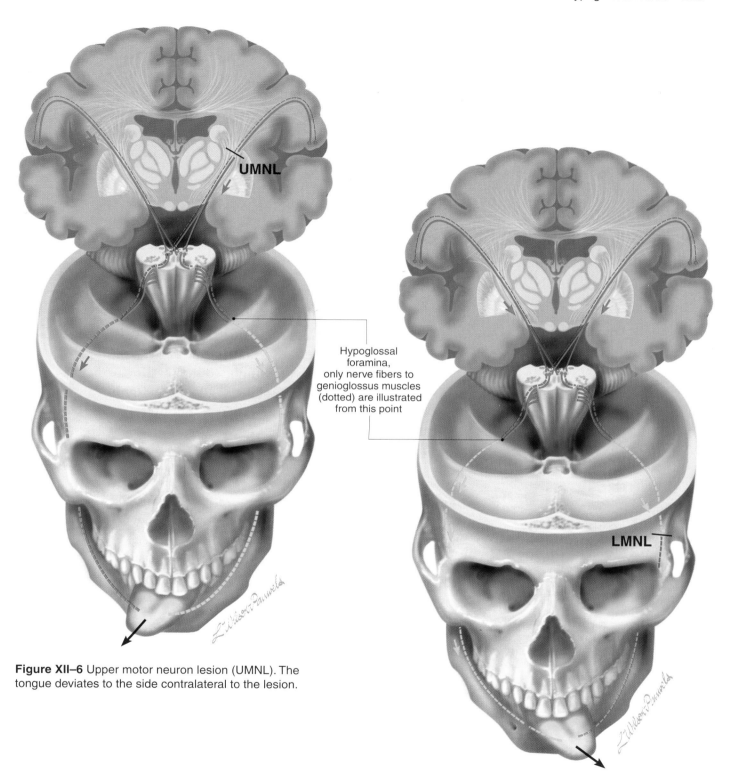

Hypoglossal
foramina,
only nerve fibers to
genioglossus muscles
(dotted) are illustrated
from this point

Figure XII–6 Upper motor neuron lesion (UMNL). The tongue deviates to the side contralateral to the lesion.

Figure XII–7 Lower motor neuron lesion (LMNL). The tongue deviates to the same side as the lesion (this is Todd's lesion).

CLINICAL TESTING

At Rest

Initially, the tongue is assessed by examining it at rest. Ask the patient to open his or her mouth, and look for evidence of fasciculations or atrophy. At rest, the tongue may deviate to the unaffected side due to the unopposed action of the styloglossus muscle that draws the tongue up and back. (See also Cranial Nerves Examination on CD-ROM.)

Protrusion

Next, ask the patient to protrude his or her tongue (Figure XII–8A). A lower motor neuron lesion will result in the tongue deviating to the ipsilateral side. The tongue deviates to the weak side because of the unopposed action of the intact contralateral genioglossus muscle. If the lesion involves upper motor neurons, the tongue will deviate to the contralateral side.

Lastly, ask the patient to push the tongue against the cheek (Figure XII–8B). If both genioglossus muscles are intact, the examiner, offering resistance by pushing on the skin of the cheek, should not be able to move the tongue to the midline from either cheek. A weakness in one of the genioglossus muscles will allow the examiner to push the tongue toward the weak side. (See also Cranial Nerves Examination on CD-ROM.)

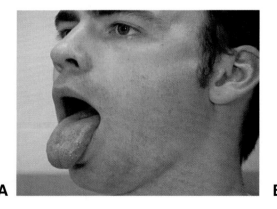 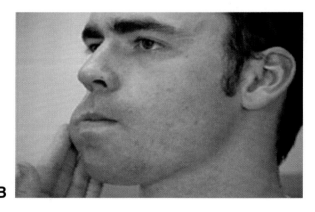

A **B**

Figure XII–8 Testing of the tongue involves *A*, protruding the tongue to observe if it sticks straight out or deviates to the side and *B*, pushing the tongue into the cheek against resistance.

ADDITIONAL RESOURCES

Brodal A. Neurological anatomy in relation to clinical medicine. 3rd ed. New York: Oxford University Press; 1981. p. 453–7.

Burt AM. Textbook of neuroanatomy. Toronto: W.B. Saunders Company Ltd.; 1993. p. 330–1.

Fitzerald MTJ. Neuroanatomy basic and clinical. 3rd ed. Toronto: W.B. Saunders Company Ltd.; 1996. p. 143–4.

Glick TH. Neurologic skills. Examination and diagnosis. New York: Blackwell Scientific Publications; 1993. p. 101.

Haines DE. Fundamental neuroscience. New York: Churchill Livingstone; 1997. p. 357.

Kiernan JA. Barr's the human nervous system. 7th ed. New York: Lippincott-Raven; 1998. p. 174–5.

Lieschke G, Davis S, Tress BM, Ebeling P. Spontaneous internal carotid artery dissection presenting as hypoglossal nerve palsy. Stroke 1988;19:1151–5.

Lindsay WK, Bone I, Callander R. Neurology and neurosurgery illustrated. 3rd ed. New York: Churchill Livingstone; 1997. p. 174–5, 181.

Martin JH. Neuroanatomy text and atlas. 2nd ed. Stamford (CT): Appleton & Lange; 1996. p. 386–9.

Moore KL, Dalley AF. Clinically oriented anatomy. 4th ed. New York: Lippincott, Williams & Wilkins; 1999. p. 862–4, 1109–10.

Nolte J. The human brain. 4th ed. Toronto: Mosby; 1999. p. 286, 288, 294.

Sturzenegger M, Huber P. Cranial nerve palsies in spontaneous carotid artery dissection. J Neurol Neurosurg Psychiatry 1993;56:1191–9.

Vighetto A, Lisovoski F, Revol A, et al. Internal carotid artery dissection and ipsilateral hypoglossal nerve palsy. J Neurol Neurosurg Psychiatry 1990;53:530–1.

13 Coordinated Eye Movements

eye movements are coordinated by reflex and voluntary neural mechanisms that influence the lower motor neurons of cranial nerves III, IV, and VI

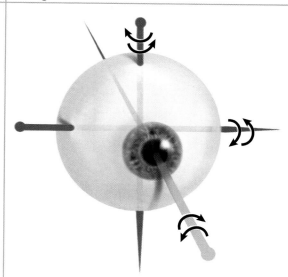

13 Coordinated Eye Movements

EYE MOVEMENTS

The human eye includes a specialized area called the fovea, which provides for high-resolution imaging and color discrimination (see Chapter II). The human oculomotor system acts to direct this specialized region toward objects of interest in the visual field and to maintain this direction. When the eye moves, the eye as a whole is not displaced. Rather, it rotates around three orthogonal axes that pass through the center of the globe (Figure 13–1). For convenience in description, eye movements are described using the cornea as a reference point. "Abduction," therefore, indicates that the cornea moves away from the nose, while "adduction" indicates that the cornea moves toward the nose. The corneas can be directed up or down in upward gaze and downward gaze. When the head is tilted laterally, the eyes rotate (intort or extort) in the opposite direction, compensating for a maximum of 40 degrees of head tilt.

Figure 13–1 depicts the six basic directions of movement. The amount that the eye can move in any one direction is limited by the attached extraocular muscles and optic nerve. Combining these movements allows the cornea to move in any direction to a maximum of 45 degrees from the relaxed position. As a rule, however, the eye does not usually move to the extremes of its range, but remains within 20 degrees of the relaxed position.

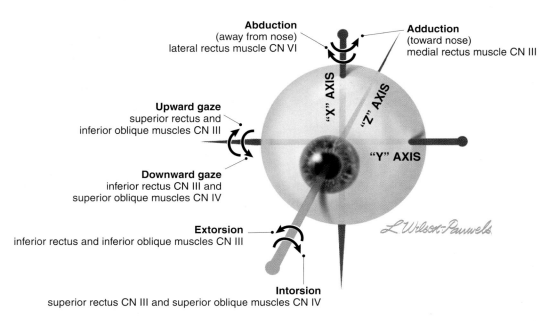

Figure 13–1 Right eye movements around the "X," "Y," and "Z" axes.

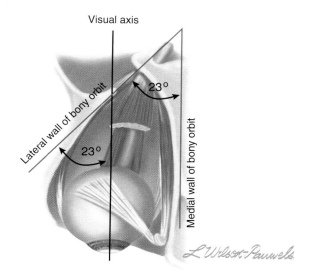

Visual axis

Lateral wall of bony orbit

23°

23°

Medial wall of bony orbit

Figure 13–2 The visual axis through the center of the cornea and fovea.

Figure 13–2 depicts the visual axis, which is an imaginary line that passes through the center of the cornea and the center of the fovea. When the eye is at rest, the visual axis is parallel to the medial wall of the bony orbit and at an angle of about 23 degrees to the lateral wall of the bony orbit.

Rotatory movements (intorsion and extorsion) are involuntary and are driven by the effects of gravity on the otolith organs in the vestibular apparatus. In space, where gravitational pull is much reduced, rotatory eye movements are thus highly compromised. Therefore, when an astronaut tilts her head, the visual field appears to slide away to the opposite side.

(Dr. Roberta Bondar, personal communication, July 2001)

The eye is moved by a total of six muscles that form three complementary, or "yoked," pairs. These pairs operate in conjunction such that when one of the muscles in the pair contracts, the other relaxes (Table 13–1).

Table 13–1 Eye Movements Produced by Cranial Nerves III, IV, and VI

Muscle	Primary Function	Secondary Function
Medial rectus (CN III)	Adduction	None
Lateral rectus (CN VI)	Abduction	None
Superior rectus (CN III)	Upward gaze	Adduction, intorsion
Inferior rectus (CN III)	Downward gaze	Adduction, extorsion
Superior oblique (CN IV)	Downward gaze	Abduction, intorsion
Inferior oblique (CN III)	Upward gaze	Abduction, extorsion

Medial and Lateral Rectus Muscles

The medial and lateral rectus muscles are involved in horizontal movement. In conjugate horizontal gaze (wherein both eyes move in the same direction by the same amount), the medial rectus muscle of one eye contracts in conjunction with the lateral rectus muscle of the other eye so that both eyes move either to the left or the right (Figures 13–3 and 13–4). At the same time, opposing muscles (ie, the yoked pair muscles) in each eye remain relaxed to allow the eyes to move freely.

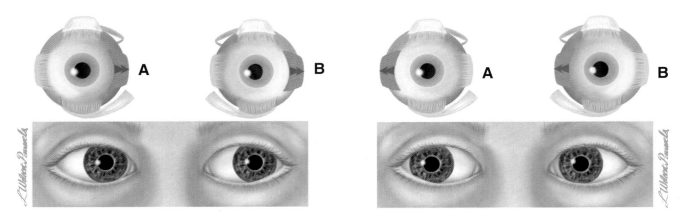

Figure 13–3 Left gaze requires the combined action of the *A*, right medial rectus muscle (CN III) and the *B*, left lateral rectus muscle (CN VI).

Figure 13–4 Right gaze requires the combined action of the *A*, right lateral rectus muscle (CN VI) and the *B*, left medial rectus muscle (CN III).

Superior and Inferior Rectus Muscles

The superior and inferior rectus muscles elevate and depress the eye, respectively, when the eye is fully abducted (away from the nose). However, when the eye is fully adducted (toward the nose), they rotate the eye about the visual axis. At intermediate eye positions, the superior and inferior rectus muscles contribute simultaneously to both vertical and rotatory movement (Figures 13–5 and 13–6).

Superior and Inferior Oblique Muscles

The superior and inferior oblique muscles depress and elevate the eye, respectively, when the eye is adducted (toward the nose), but they rotate the eye about the visual axis when the eye is abducted (away from the nose). At eye positions between fully abducted and fully adducted, the superior and inferior oblique muscles contribute to both vertical and rotatory movement (Figures 13–7 and 13–8). When the eye is looking straight ahead, the superior and inferior rectus muscles and the superior and inferior oblique muscles each contribute about 50 percent of the vertical and rotatory movement.

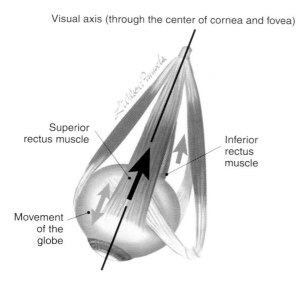

Figure 13–5 Superior and inferior rectus muscles in abduction. When the right eye is abducted, the PULL (*black and grey arrows*) exerted by the superior and inferior rectus muscles is parallel to the visual axis. Therefore, the superior and inferior rectus muscles **elevate** and **depress** the eye, respectively (*orange arrow*). Both are innervated by cranial nerve III.

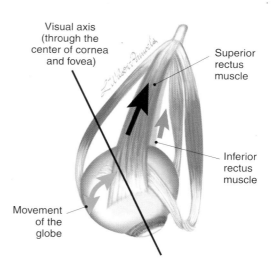

Figure 13–6 Superior and inferior rectus muscles in adduction. When the right eye is adducted, the PULL (*black and grey arrows*) exerted by the superior and inferior rectus muscles is at an angle to the visual axis. Therefore, the superior and inferior rectus muscles **intort** and **extort** the eye, respectively (*orange arrow*). Both are innervated by cranial nerve III.

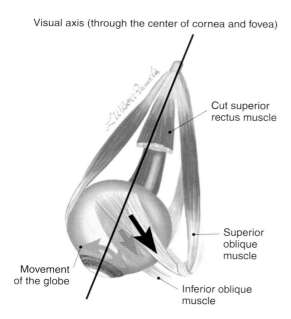

Figure 13–7 Superior and inferior oblique muscles in abduction. When the right eye is abducted the PULL (*black and grey arrows*) exerted by superior and inferior oblique muscles is at an angle to the visual axis. Therefore, the superior (cranial nerve IV) and inferior (cranial nerve III) oblique muscles **intort** and **extort** the eye, respectively (*orange arrow*).

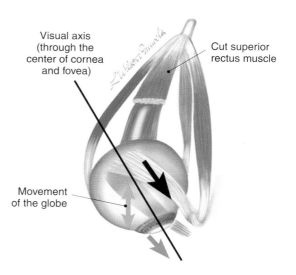

Figure 13–8 Superior and inferior oblique muscles in adduction. When the right eye is adducted the PULL (*black and grey arrows*) exerted by the superior and inferior oblique muscles is parallel to the visual axis. Therefore, the superior (cranial nerve IV) and inferior (cranial nerve III) oblique muscles **depress** and **elevate** the eye, respectively (*orange arrow*).

TYPES OF EYE MOVEMENTS

- *Smooth pursuit* movements keep an object of interest imaged on the fovea when either the head, the object, or both are moving.
- *Saccades* are rapid eye movements that change visual fixation to a new object of interest.
- *Nystagmus* is an oscillatory movement in which smooth pursuit movements and saccades alternate. Nystagmus can be normal (see below) or, in the absence of an appropriate stimulus, can signal pathology.
- *Conjugate* (together) movement is when both eyes move in the same direction by the same amount.
- *Vergent or disconjugate* (convergent or divergent) movement is when the eyes move in opposite directions (ie, they converge or diverge for near and far vision, respectively).

There are five neural mechanisms that control eye movements:

- Vestibulo-ocular reflex (VOR)
- Optokinetic reflex (OKR)
- Pursuit system
- Saccadic system
- Vergence system

> Some authors describe a sixth oculomotor mechanism that maintains visual fixation. Since the elasticity of the ocular tissues tends to pull the eye to a neutral position (ie, straight ahead in the orbit), muscle activity is required to maintain eye position in any other direction. The pathways that subserve this mechanism are not well understood in humans, and will not be addressed here.

Vestibulo-ocular Reflex

The function of the VOR is to move the eyes to compensate for movements of the head, such that visual fixation on a chosen object can be maintained. The vestibular apparatus (Chapter VIII) provides the sensory signals that drive the VOR. Head movement stimulates the sensory receptors in the vestibular apparatus, which, in turn, signal the vestibular nuclei in the floor of the fourth ventricle. The vestibular nuclei (predominantly the medial subnuclei) signal the lower motor neurons in the abducens, trochlear, and oculomotor nuclei. Signals are also sent from the vestibular nucleus to the internuclear neurons in the abducens nucleus, which, in turn, project rostrally via the medial longitudinal fasciculus (MLF) to the lower motor neurons of cranial nerve III that innervate the contralateral medial rectus muscle (Figure 13–9). In this way, the lower motor neurons drive the extraocular muscles to produce appropriate compensatory eye movements. The vestibulocerebellum, the

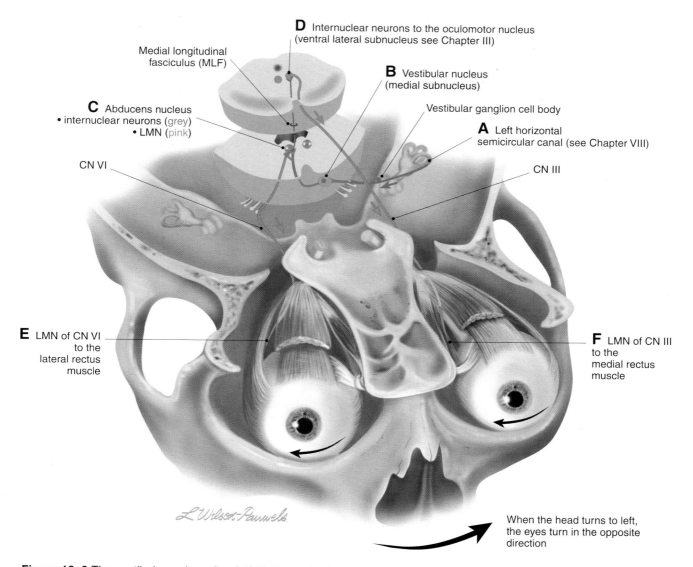

Figure 13–9 The vestibulo-ocular reflex (VOR) illustrating horizontal eye movement only. The excitatory pathway is from the *A*, left horizontal semicircular canal to the *B*, vestibular nucleus to the lower motor neurons (LMN) of *C*, cranial nerve VI nuclei and *D*, cranial nerve III nuclei (via the medial longitudinal fasciculus from the abducens nucleus) to the *E*, right lateral and *F*, left medial rectus muscles, respectively.

interstitial nucleus of Cajal, and the nucleus prepositus hypoglossi help to further coordinate this movement.

The VOR is particularly important in maintaining visual fixation during locomotion. The frequency of head movements during locomotion is on the order of 0.5 to 5.0 cycles per second. These movements require relatively rapid compensatory eye movements. Because transduction in the vestibular apparatus takes very little time (a few microseconds), the VOR is able to respond to changes in head movement quickly. If the VOR is compromised, visual acuity during locomotion degrades significantly. Under conditions of sustained head rotation, the eyes counter-rotate smoothly and then snap back to a neutral position in the orbit and begin a new smooth pursuit movement in the same direction as the original one. This alternating smooth pursuit–saccadic movement is called vestibular nystagmus.

The VOR adapts rapidly. When head rotation is sustained, the fluid in the semicircular canals accelerates to match the speed of the head, and the sensory signal degrades. In these conditions, a second system of maintaining visual fixation, the optokinetic reflex, becomes important.

Optokinetic Reflex

The OKR is similar to the vestibulo-ocular reflex in that it generates a smooth pursuit movement that is equal in velocity but opposite in direction to the movement of the head. A smooth pursuit movement tracks the passing visual field for a distance and then a saccade brings the eyes back to a neutral position, and a new smooth pursuit movement is generated to follow the visual field again. This oscillating eye movement is called optokinetic nystagmus (OKN). A familiar example of optokinetic nystagmus is the movements of the eyes as they follow the passing scenery from a moving vehicle.

The sensory signals that drive the OKR arise in the retina. Because visual processing in the retina is slow relative to signal transduction in the semicircular canals, the OKR responds slowly to changes in the movement of the visual fields across the retina. However, unlike the VOR, it does not adapt, which means that the sensory signals that drive the reflex do not degrade with time. Retinal ganglion cell axons enter the optic nerve and project caudally to the pretectal region of the midbrain, which also receives signals from the visual association areas of the occipital lobes. In turn, the pretectal region projects to the vestibular nucleus (mainly the medial subnucleus) in the medulla by presently unknown pathways. The medial subnucleus projects to the lower motor neurons in the abducens, trochlear, and oculomotor nuclei and also to the internuclear neurons in the abducens nucleus (Figure 13–10).

Pursuit System

The pursuit system generates the eye movements involved in following a moving object against a stationary background (ie, following a butterfly in a garden). Since this system acts to keep moving images centered on the fovea, it follows that only animals with a fovea have a smooth pursuit system.

Signals for voluntary pursuit arise in the extrastriate visual cortex of the temporal lobe. The precise route by which these signals reach the lower motor neurons is not known with certainty. However, it seems likely to follow a progression where the extrastriate cortex signals the dorsolateral pontine nuclei in the pons, which, in turn, signal the flocculus and posterior vermis of the cerebellum, which signal the vestibular nucleus (mainly the medial subnucleus) that projects via the MLF to the nuclei of cranial nerves III, IV, and VI.

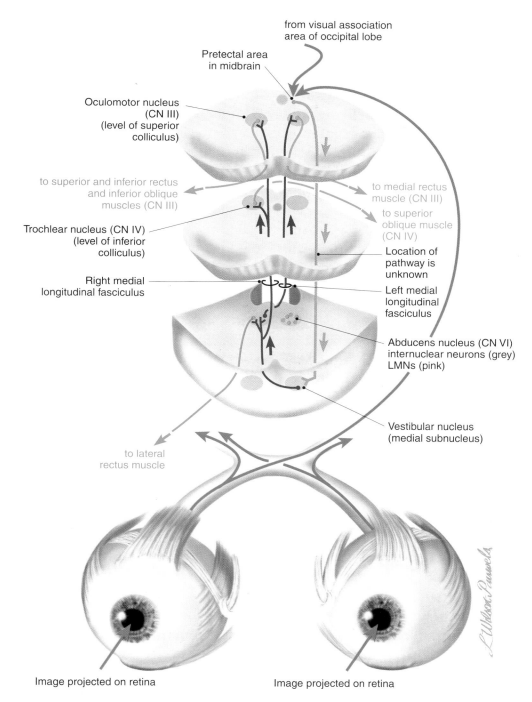

from visual association
area of occipital lobe

Pretectal area
in midbrain

Oculomotor nucleus
(CN III)
(level of superior
colliculus)

to superior and inferior rectus
and inferior oblique
muscles (CN III)

to medial rectus
muscle (CN III)

to superior
oblique muscle
(CN IV)

Trochlear nucleus (CN IV)
(level of inferior
colliculus)

Location of
pathway is
unknown

Right medial
longitudinal fasciculus

Left medial
longitudinal
fasciculus

Abducens nucleus (CN VI)
internuclear neurons (grey)
LMNs (pink)

Vestibular nucleus
(medial subnucleus)

to lateral
rectus muscle

Image projected on retina

Image projected on retina

Figure 13–10 The optokinetic reflex (OKR). Excitatory pathway shown for right gaze only.
LMNs = lower motor neurons.

Saccadic System

The saccadic system shifts the fovea rapidly from one target to another, moving the eyes at speeds of up to 900 degrees per second. The high speed of saccadic movement minimizes the time that the fovea is off target. Signals for saccadic movement arise in the superior colliculi in the midbrain. The superior colliculi receive saccade-generating signals from four major sources: the frontal eye fields of the frontal lobes, which are involved in consciously selecting an object of interest; the retinae; the somatosensory system; and the auditory system (Figure 13–11).

The saccades generated by the frontal eye fields are the only totally voluntary eye movements that we make. The saccades generated in response to signals from the retinae, the somatosensory system, and the auditory system are visual reflexes. For example, we reflexively orient our eyes to a sudden flash of light, a loud sound, or an area of the body that is subjected to unexpected (usually noxious) sensory input.

Gaze Centers

The frontal eye fields and the superior colliculi project to "gaze centers" in the reticular formation of the brain stem. Two gaze centers have been identified: one for vertical gaze (the rostral interstitial nucleus of the MLF) and one for lateral gaze (the paramedian pontine reticular formation). These reticular nuclei project to the nuclei of nerves III, IV, and VI, which, in turn, generate saccades that redirect the fovea to an appropriate location. They are also responsible for the saccadic phase of the optokinetic reflex and vestibulo-ocular nystagmus.

Vergence System

The four eye movement systems described previously produce conjugate movements (ie, both eyes move in the same direction by the same amount). In contrast, the vergence system moves the eyes in opposing directions, usually by differing amounts. The vergence system is present only in animals with binocular vision and is part of the accommodation reflex (see Chapter III).

When attention is shifted from one object to another object that is closer or further away, the eyes converge or diverge until the image occupies the same relative location on both retinae and only one image is perceived. For the eyes to converge (see Chapter III, Figure III–8), both medial rectus muscles are activated and both lateral rectus muscles are inhibited. For divergence, the opposite set of muscle actions is necessary. Little is known about the precise location of a "vergence" center in humans. However, it is likely in the midbrain, close to the oculomotor nucleus.

The vergence system works in conjunction with the smooth pursuit and saccadic systems. The sensory stimulus for vergence is disparity between the relative locations of the images on both retinae. This disparity is detected by extrastriate visual cortex neurons, which presumably project to the vergence center in the midbrain.

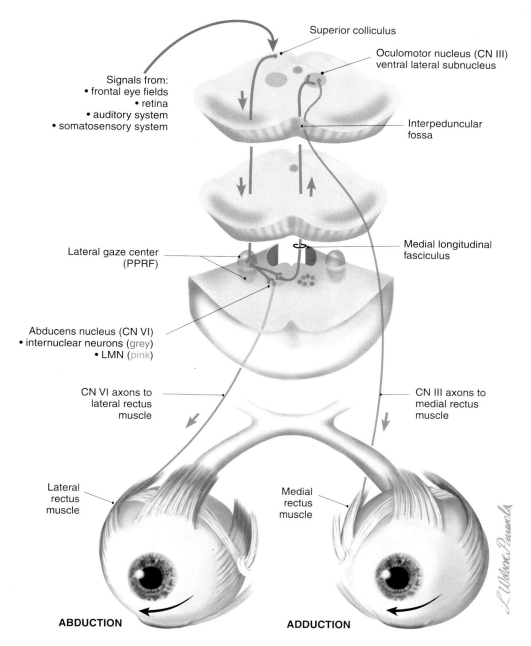

Superior colliculus

Oculomotor nucleus (CN III)
ventral lateral subnucleus

Signals from:
• frontal eye fields
• retina
• auditory system
• somatosensory system

Interpeduncular
fossa

Lateral gaze center
(PPRF)

Medial longitudinal
fasciculus

Abducens nucleus (CN VI)
• internuclear neurons (grey)
• LMN (pink)

CN VI axons to
lateral rectus
muscle

CN III axons to
medial rectus
muscle

Lateral
rectus
muscle

Medial
rectus
muscle

ABDUCTION

ADDUCTION

Figure 13–11 The saccadic system—the pathway for right lateral gaze. PPRF = paramedian
pontine reticular formation.

Internuclear Ophthalmoplegia

Internuclear ophthalmoplegia is characterized by paresis of adduction in one eye and horizontal nystagmus in the contralateral abducting eye. This is due to a lesion in the MLF on the side of the adducting eye. With right lateral gaze, a lesion in the left MLF results in failure of adduction in the left eye and horizontal nystagmus in the right eye (Figure 13–12). Paresis of the medial rectus muscle can be caused by damage to its lower motor neurons or to the pathways in the MLF that activate the lower motor neurons (internuclear ophthalmoplegia). If the medial rectus muscle cannot be activated by attempted lateral gaze, but can be activated by attempted convergence, then the lesion is likely in the MLF (see Figure 13–12). Internuclear ophthalmoplegia can be monocular or binocular depending on whether the MLF is affected on one side or on both sides.

CLINICAL TESTING

To test eye movements, draw a large "H" in the air a few feet in front of the patient and ask him or her to follow your finger with his or her eyes. The horizontal bar of the "H" will test medial and lateral rectus muscles. The two vertical bars of the "H" will isolate and test the motion of the superior or inferior rectus muscles and the inferior or superior oblique muscles (Figure 13–13). The eyes should move in a smooth, coordinated motion throughout the "H." (See also Cranial Nerves Examination on CD-ROM.)

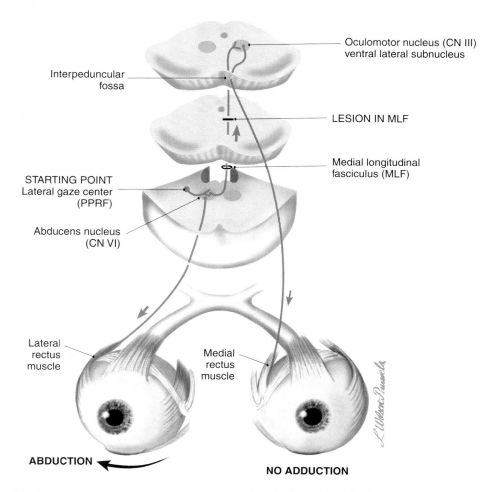

Oculomotor nucleus (CN III)
ventral lateral subnucleus

Interpeduncular
fossa

LESION IN MLF

Medial longitudinal
fasciculus (MLF)

STARTING POINT
Lateral gaze center
(PPRF)

Abducens nucleus
(CN VI)

Lateral
rectus
muscle

Medial
rectus
muscle

ABDUCTION

NO ADDUCTION

Figure 13–12 Internuclear ophthalmoplegia caused by a lesion of the MLF between the abducens and midbrain nuclei. Follow the pathway starting at the lateral gaze center. PPRF = paramedian pontine reticular formation.

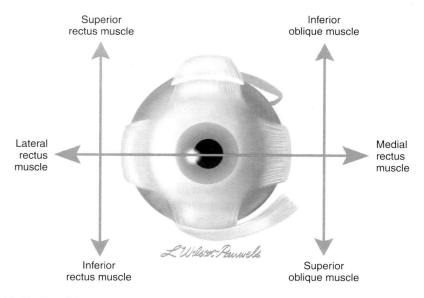

Superior
rectus muscle

Inferior
oblique muscle

Lateral
rectus
muscle

Medial
rectus
muscle

Inferior
rectus muscle

Superior
oblique muscle

Figure 13–13 Testing right eye movements.

ADDITIONAL RESOURCES

Brodal A. Neurological anatomy in relation to clinical medicine. 3rd ed. New York: Oxford University Press; 1981. p. 532–77.

Büttner U, Büttner-Ennever JA. Present concepts of oculomotor organization. In: Büttner-Ennever JA, editor. Neuroanatomy of the oculomotor system. Amsterdam: Elsevier; 1988. p. 3–32.

Glimcher PA. Eye movements. In: Zigmond MJ, Bloom FE, Landis SC, et al, editors. Fundamental neuroscience. San Diego: Academic Press; 1999. p. 993–1009.

Goldberg MW. The control of gaze. In: Kandel ER, Schwartz JH, Jessell TM, editors. Principles of neural science. 4th ed. New York: McGraw Hill; 2000. p. 782–800.

Goldberg ME, Hudspeth AJ. The vestibular system. In: Kandel ER, Schwartz JH, Jessell TM, editors. Principles of neural science. 4th ed. New York: McGraw Hill; 2000. p. 801–15.

Leigh RJ, Zee DS. The neurology of eye movements. 3rd ed. New York: Oxford University Press; 1999. p. 3–15.

Stahl JS. Eye-head coordination and the variation of eye-movement accuracy with orbital eccentricity. Exp Brain Res 2001;136:200–10.

Index